The Principles and Practice of Physical Therapy

by

William Arnould-Taylor

MSc PhD (Physiology)

3rd EDITION

Stanley Thornes (Publishers) Ltd

First published in 1977 for
Arnould-Taylor Education Ltd.
2nd Edition 1982
Reprinted 1983
Reprinted 1984 with minor corrections
Reprinted 1986
Reprinted 1988
Reprinted 1989
3rd Edition 1991
by
Stanley Thornes (Publishers) Ltd
Ellenborough House
Wellington Street
Cheltenham GL50 1YD
UK

Reprinted 1992
Reprinted 1993
Reprinted 1994
Reprinted 1995

ISBN 0 7487 1250 X

Companion volumes to this title
THE AESTHETICIENNE by Ann Hagman
A TEXTBOOK OF HOLISTIC AROMATHERAPY by W. Arnould-Taylor
A TEXTBOOK OF ANATOMY AND PHYSIOLOGY by W. Arnould Taylor
and
Aileen Harris
PRINCIPLES AND PRACTICE OF PERFUMERY AND COSMETICS
by G. Howard and W. Arnould-Taylor

Photoset in Linotron Sabon with Univers
by Northern Phototypesetting Co. Ltd, Bolton, Lancashire
Printed and bound at Redwood Books, Wiltshire

Contents

Part I The Study of Anatomy and Physiology:

		page
Chapter 1	**Introduction to Anatomy and Physiology**	3
Chapter 2	**The Skeletal System**	8
Chapter 3	**The Muscular System**	19
Chapter 4	**The Vascular System**	30
Chapter 5	**The Neurological System**	40
Chapter 6	**The Digestive System**	51
Chapter 7	**The Respiratory System**	59
Chapter 8	**The Genito-Urinary System**	65
Chapter 9	**The Endocrine System**	72
Chapter 10	**Accessory Organs**	77
Chapter 11	**Histology**	85

Part II The Study and Application of Therapy Treatments:

Chapter 12	**Massage**	97
	(a) Swedish	
	(b) Oil	
	(c) Mechanical	
Chapter 13	**Sauna, Steam and other Hydrotherapy Treatments**	112
Chapter 14	**Vacuum Suction Treatments**	121
Chapter 15	**Electricity in Treatment**	129
	(a) General	
	(b) Faradism	
	(c) Galvanism	
Chapter 16	**Ultraviolet and Infrared Rays**	143
Chapter 17	**Exercises**	150
	(a) Manual	
	(b) Mechanical	

Chapter 18   **Other Forms of Treatment:**   156
              (a)   High Frequency
              (b)   Diapulse
              (c)   Short Wave
              (d)   Microwave
              (e)   Interferential

Chapter 19   **First-aid**   161

Part III **Specialised Aspects of Physical Therapy:**

Chapter 20   **Sports Therapy**   167
Chapter 21   **Ultrasound**   175

Part IV **Management of Patient and Practice:**

Chapter 22   **Patient Assessment**   189
Chapter 23   **Clinic Organisation and Management**   193
Chapter 24   **Professionalism, Ethics and Patient Support** 205
              Conclusion   209
              Some Useful Addresses   210
              Index   211

Foreword

The *raison d'être* for this textbook is a simple one. Having spent many years teaching the subjects of Anatomy, Physiology and Physical Therapy, and examining up to 1000 students a year—I was acutely conscious of the absence of a book which combined the subjects in a single volume. Having been urged by many medical and para-medical friends to write such a book I have at last succumbed to their insistent 'badgering' and the following pages are the consequence.

I am aware that in a composite volume, which has of necessity to be kept to a reasonable textbook size, there are bound to be omissions and deficiencies. I hope however that the particular format which I have employed will make a study of the subjects interesting and inspire readers to pursue their learning in greater depth.

I wish to place on record my appreciation of the help given by Miss Kim Solly M.Phys., L.C.S.P. in reading the proofs and for her many helpful suggestions which have been incorporated in the text wherever practical.

Also thanks to the illustrators from Oxford Illustrators Ltd., for their accurate interpretation of my wishes.

William Arnould-Taylor   10.9.76

Preface to 1991 Edition

The Anatomy and Physiology section of this textbook is little altered from the first edition. The basic format followed allows for little change, the greatest developments being in microbiology and immunology—fields generally outside the scope of this book.

On the other hand, physical treatments and our evaluation of their efficiency are constantly changing so the second part of the book has been the subject of a number of deletions and additions in an effort to enable the student to keep abreast of current trends.

Also on the suggestion of the publishers two new sections have been added enlarging the scope of the book to encompass problems created by the ever increasing interest in leisure activities.

Again, I am grateful to my colleague, Kim Aldridge M.Phys., for her assistance both in proof reading and helpful suggestions.

WILLIAM ARNOULD-TAYLOR
Oakelbrook Mill
Newent
Glos GL18 1HD

Part I
The Study of Anatomy and Physiology

Chapter 1

Introduction to Anatomy and Physiology

A review of standard textbooks on anatomy and physiology reveals that the majority are written with the medical student or nurse particularly in mind and few—if any—have been written specifically for the physical therapist. The result is that the physical therapist often has to wade through a good deal of material which is going to be largely valueless to him/her in the practice of the profession. The difference of approach between, say, a nurse on the one hand and a physical therapist on the other, is a basic one—the nurse is primarily concerned with what happens inside the body, that is beneath the skin, whereas the physical therapist is more concerned with the exterior of the body and those parts of the body which may be influenced from the exterior.

It has been found that very detailed textbooks on anatomy and physiology, though excellent for medical and nursing students, leave other students a little confused as to what is most suitable for them to select for the purposes of their studies. It is hoped, therefore, that this comparatively small section on anatomy and physiology will help to fill the gap. It makes no pretence of enveloping the whole of the subject matter of anatomy and physiology but aims to give the student a basic understanding of the relative parts of the body and their functions.

First of all the student should have a clear understanding of the difference between the two terms—anatomy and physiology. Anatomy is normally defined as being the study of the structure of the body and the relationship of various parts one to another; whereas physiology is the study of the functions of those parts. For example—to say that the human heart is approximately 255 g in weight, is somewhat pear-shaped in appearance and lies two-thirds to the left-hand side of the rib cage and one-third to the right, is to describe its anatomy; that is its weight, shape and position. On the other hand, this information tells us nothing at all about the function of the heart so we have to look at the physiology to learn that the heart is basically a pump which forces oxygenated blood around the body and, at the same time, circulates the venous or carbon dioxide loaded blood around the lungs for reoxygenisation. Therefore, by combining the knowledge of anatomy and physiology of the heart we are able to get a picture of what it looks like as well as what it does. In the ensuing chapters anatomy and physiology are dealt with together.

For the purpose of simplicity of learning—the body is divided into eight systems. In some textbooks these basic systems are sub-divided so that nine, ten or more systems are quoted. However, on closer investigation, it will be seen that these additional systems are really part of the basic systems. These we divide as follows:

(1) *The skeletal system* which, as its name implies, is the bony structure on which the other systems depend for support.
(2) *The muscular system.*
(3) *The vascular system* which includes the lymphatic system.
(4) *The neurological system* which covers all the nerves of the body as well as the brain.

These four systems we refer to as the *major systems*—not because they are more important than the systems which follow—but because they are the systems which envelop the whole of the body and are the ones which can most easily be affected by the professional skills of the physical therapist.

We now pass on to:

(5) *The digestive system.*
(6) *The respiratory system.*
(7) *The genito-urinary system* which includes the reproductive and kidney systems.
(8) *The endocrine system.*

These last four systems are referred to as the *minor systems*.

All professions have their own peculiar vocabularies—these are necessary for the accurate understanding of the subject matter— and the profession of medicine is no exception. It has a very wide vocabulary which requires a lifetime to master fully. There are, however, parts of this vocabulary which are essential to the physical therapist and these are dealt with in the form of a glossary at the end of each chapter so as not to interfere with the flow of the text of the lesson itself. The attention of students is, however, specially directed to the necessity of understanding this terminology because if the words are learnt in relation to the appropriate discussion it makes the subsequent learning that much easier.

HISTORY

It is not possible to trace the beginnings of the study of anatomy and physiology for these are lost in antiquity. The ancient Egyptians were famous for their embalming processes which must have involved a certain amount of knowledge of the anatomy of the human body and they had a system of medicine— traces of which survive until today. The *R* which a doctor writes at the top of his prescription is, in fact, the 'R' symbol for the Eye of Horus—the hawk-headed sun god who lost his eye in battle and had it restored by Thoth, the patron god of physicians. Thoth was one of the many gods invoked by doctors of ancient Egypt when administering their remedies.

About the same time, but in an entirely different part of the world, the Chinese were practising a form of medicine, acupuncture, which involved some 365 different needling points, but it is to the civilisation of the Greek period that we have to look for more detailed knowledge of human anatomy.

From this era we have the work of Hippocrates, who is often referred to as the father of medicine, and, in a rather different role, the name of Aristotle, who is generally acknowledged as being the founder of comparative anatomy.

During the Roman period which followed there was a medical school in Rome and the fine selection of surgical and dissecting instruments which have been preserved indicates a considerable knowledge of the structure of the human body.

Galen lived in the second century and his name is still remembered as being that of one of the greatest physicians and anatomists of antiquity. His work formed the basis of the European knowledge of anatomy for well over a thousand years, surviving through the Dark Ages into the Middle Ages when we see the beginning of the great Italian medical schools and universities such as Bologna and Padua. One of the 16th century graduates was Paracelsus von Hohenheim, a progressive medical teacher, who did much to alter the accepted ideas of his day. It was in 1543 that Versalius published his first drawings of the structure of the human body and so paved the way for modern anatomy. Nearly a hundred years later, in 1628, Harvey announced his discovery of the role of the heart in the circulation of the blood through the lungs and the body, and in 1661 Malpighi discovered the capillary circulation and so completed the knowledge of how blood from arteries is returned to the heart by way of veins.

In the middle of the 18th century Auenbrugger of Austria invented percussion—a method by which doctors could diagnose the condition of the lungs. As a boy he had often watched his father tap barrels to see how much wine they contained and he applied the same technique to the chests of his patients. If they gave out hollow sounds similar to those of empty barrels he considered they were healthy whilst a muffled or high-pitched note indicated the presence of some unhealthy fluid.

At the end of the 18th century—1798—Jenner discovered that vaccination could be employed as a preventive of smallpox. Early in the 19th century the French physician, Rene Laennec, invented the stethoscope. He was attending a patient suffering from heart disease and, as she was rather obese, he decided that applying an ear direct to the chest (which was the usual method) would be of little use. He remembered that children sometimes amused themselves by playing with logs of wood, one child making tapping or scratching noises at one end and the other one listening at the other. So he rolled up a cylinder of paper and put one end of the stethoscope to the patient's chest and his ear to the other and found that he could hear the heart beating much more clearly than before. He then experimented with other materials until the stethoscope was invented.

The first real knowledge of the digestive system came in 1822 when a man by the name of Alexis St. Martin was wounded in the stomach in a brawl near Lake Michigan. He recovered but the wound left a permanent hole through which Dr William Beaumont, U.S. Army, was able to watch how the stomach exuded the juices needed for digestion.

In the 1840s nitrous oxide or laughing gas was first used by a dentist in America for the extraction of teeth. This was quickly followed by the use of ether in hospital operating theatres which made possible a much more detailed study of anatomy. In 1867 Lister established the principles of antisepsis and in 1877 Pasteur demonstrated the role of germs in the causation of disease. In 1895 Röntgen discovered X-rays and in 1898 the Curies isolated radium. In 1904 Bayliss and Starling identified the first hormone. 1912 saw the discovery of vitamins by Frederick Gowland Hopkins whilst in 1928 Alexander Fleming discovered the antibiotic—penicillin—though this was not to come into medical use until about 1939.

Anatomy and physiology are subjects of continuous research and discovery and all the knowledge which we have accumulated in this century serves to indicate that we are only at the beginning of a complete understanding of these two subjects.

GLOSSARY

Some general terms used in Anatomy and
Physiology.

The Anatomical Position an erect position of the human body with arms by
sides and palms of the hands facing forward

Anterior applies to the front of the body when in the erect
position

Distal the opposite of proximal and the part furthest away
from the median line; so distal thigh will be at the
knee end of the thigh

Dorsal synonymous with posterior; normally used when
describing the hand or the foot

Lateral either side of the median line, e.g. the outer side of the
arm will be its lateral aspect whilst the inner side is
described as the medial aspect

Median Line an imaginary line which runs through the centre of
the body from the centre of the crown of the head
ending up directly between the two feet

Morphology the study of differences and resemblances in structure
and form

Posterior the back of the body when in the erect position

Proximal a term of comparison applied to structures which are
nearer the centre of the body or the median line, e.g.
proximal thigh is the end of the thigh nearest to the
centre of the body

Symmetrical similar parts of the body, e.g. right and left ears, eyes,
tibias, or limbs

Chapter 2

The Skeletal System

The skeleton provides the framework of the body and it has two principal functions. The first is that of *protection*, for example:

the skull protects the brain,

the rib cage protects principally the heart and the lungs,

the spinal column protects the spinal cord,

the pelvic bones provide a certain amount of protection for the viscera.

The second function is that of *locomotion* or *movement*.

The skeleton is made up of 206 bones though this figure varies slightly in different textbooks due to the fact that some authorities count the number of bones which are present in a young child whereas other authorities consider that only the bones of an adult should be counted, as by the time adulthood is reached certain childhood bones will have fused together.

Bone is a dry dense tissue composed of approximately 25 per cent water, 30 per cent organic material and 45 per cent mineral. The mineral matter consists chiefly of calcium phosphate and a small amount of magnesium salts; these give the bone its rigidity and hardness. The organic matter consists of fibrous material which gives the bone its toughness and resilience. There are five classifications of bone:

(1) **Long bones** e.g. the femur or thigh bone, the longest and strongest bone of the body.

(2) **Short bones** e.g. metatarsal bones.

(3) **Flat bones** e.g. frontal bone of the head.

(4) **Irregular bones** e.g. the vertebrae.

(5) **Sesamoid bones**—rounded masses found in certain tendons of muscles, the best example being the patella or knee cap.

A long bone normally consists of marrow surrounded by a spongy bone layer which, in turn, is surrounded by a compact bone layer and finally by a hard outside covering known as the periosteum.

In addition to the two principal functions of the skeleton, individual bones serve other purposes such as the attachment of tendons and muscles, and the formation of red blood cells and some white blood cells in the bone marrow.

A *joint* is formed where two bones meet. Joints may be divided according to their mobility, into three types:

THE SKELETON

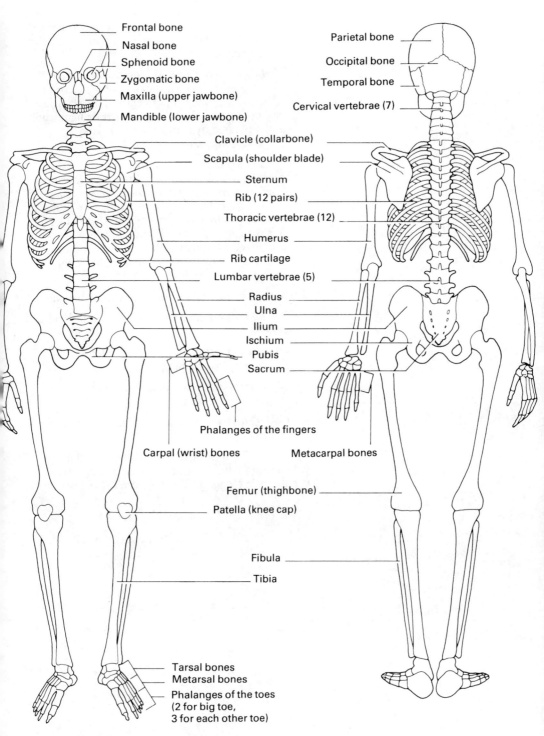

Frontal bone
Nasal bone
Sphenoid bone
Zygomatic bone
Maxilla (upper jawbone)
Mandible (lower jawbone)

Parietal bone
Occipital bone
Temporal bone
Cervical vertebrae (7)

Clavicle (collarbone)
Scapula (shoulder blade)
Sternum
Rib (12 pairs)
Thoracic vertebrae (12)
Humerus
Rib cartilage
Lumbar vertebrae (5)
Radius
Ulna
Ilium
Ischium
Pubis
Sacrum

Phalanges of the fingers

Carpal (wrist) bones   Metacarpal bones

Femur (thighbone)
Patella (knee cap)

Fibula

Tibia

Tarsal bones
Metarsal bones
Phalanges of the toes
(2 for big toe,
3 for each other toe)

(1) *Fixed joints or synarthroses* provide no movement, for example the sutures between the skull bones. There is fibrous tissue between the bones, which either overlap or are fitted together in a jagged line.

(2) *Slightly movable joints or amphiathroses* are found in the pelvis (*symphysis pubis*), sacro-iliac joint and the joints at both ends of the clavicle. The bones are held together by strong ligaments and separated by pads of fibrocartilage (*cartilaginous joints*).

(3) *Freely movable joints* are enclosed in a fibrous capsule, supported by ligaments. This capsule is lined by a *synovial membrane* with *synovial fluid* in the cavity. This is a whitish fluid, not unlike raw egg-white in consistency, which acts like oil in a machine to reduce friction between the articulating surfaces of the joint. The bone surfaces are covered by *hyaline* cartilage for smoother operation.

There are four main groups of freely movable joints:

(a) *Ball and socket articulations*—hip joint, shoulder joint

(b) *Hinge articulations*—knee joint (full hinge), elbow joint (partial hinge)

(c) *Pivot articulations*—radius and ulna joints, axis joint of cervical spine

(d) *Gliding joints*—tarsal joint of ankle, carpal joint of wrist.

The knee joint is the only articulation in the body which forms a full hinge, that is, the bones are capable of moving in either forward or backward

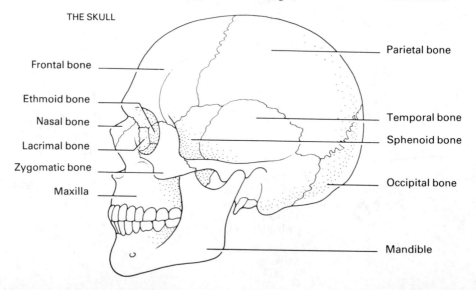

THE SKULL

Frontal bone

Ethmoid bone

Nasal bone

Lacrimal bone

Zygomatic bone

Maxilla

Parietal bone

Temporal bone

Sphenoid bone

Occipital bone

Mandible

directions. In practice this is prevented by the patella or kneecap which fits into the hinge rather like a doorstop or wedge. When the patella is not present, for example when it has been broken in an accident, the lower leg comes forward.

The capsule of the freely movable joints possesses small sacs containing a clear, viscous fluid. These structures which are called *mucous bursae* secrete synovial fluid. If the synovial membrane becomes inflamed this is known as *synovitis*, a well known example being tennis elbow. If the bursae become inflamed this is known as *bursitis*; the best known example of this is housemaid's knee—an occupational hazard for people whose work involves a good deal of kneeling.

Distribution of Bones in the Skeleton

22 bones form the skull bones, 8 of the cranium:

1 frontal bone forming the forehead
2 parietal bones forming the top and sides of the cranium
1 occipital bone
2 temporal bones
1 sphenoid bone
1 ethmoid bone

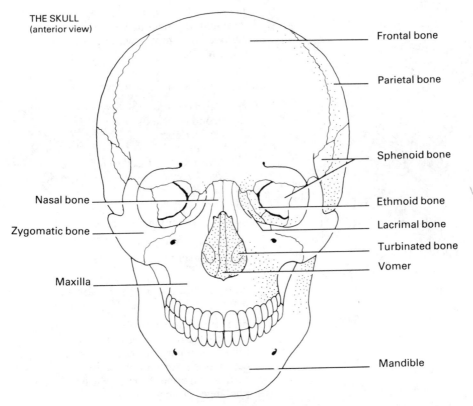

THE SKULL
(anterior view)

Frontal bone

Parietal bone

Sphenoid bone

Nasal bone

Ethmoid bone

Zygomatic bone

Lacrimal bone

Turbinated bone

Vomer

Maxilla

Mandible

and 14 bones of the face—of which the principal bones are:

the superior maxilla or upper jaw
the mandible or lower jaw (the jawbone which moves)
2 zygomatic or cheek bones
2 nasal bones which form the bridge of the nose
2 lacrimal bones.

25 bones form the thorax (or chest):

the sternum or breast bone
12 pairs of ribs.

The first 7 pairs are known as *true ribs* because each rib is joined to the sternum directly. The next 5 pairs (8—12th) are known as *false ribs* because they do not join the sternum directly. The 8th, 9th and 10th ribs fuse with the rib immediately above, while the 11th and 12th pairs (*floating ribs*) only partly surround the circumference of the thorax and are unattached in front.

33 bones form the spine:

24 *true* or *movable* vertebrae, separated by pads of fibrocartilage
9 *false or fixed* vertebrae, closely fused together with no movement between them except the coccyx which moves with respect to the sacrum.

From the top of the spine downwards there are:

7 cervical vertebrae—the first is the atlas bone, the second is the axis bone
12 thoracic vertebrae
5 lumbar vertebrae
5 sacral vertebrae—fused to form the sacrum
4 coccygeal vertebrae—fused to form the coccyx.

4 bones form the shoulder girdle:

2 clavicles or collar bones
2 scapulae or shoulder blades.

60 bones form the upper limbs, 30 bones in each whole arm:

1 humerus or upper arm
1 radius—the outer bone of the forearm
1 ulna—the inner bone of the forearm
8 carpal bones forming the wrist
5 metacarpal bones forming the hand, and
14 phalanges or finger bones.

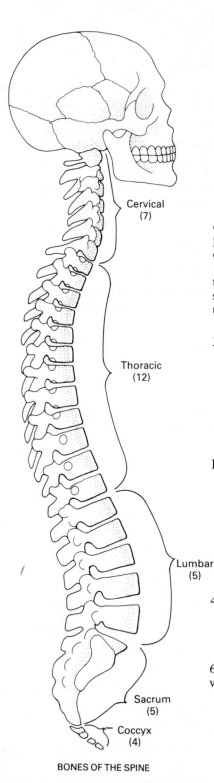

Cervical (7)

Thoracic (12)

Lumbar (5)

Sacrum (5)

Coccyx (4)

BONES OF THE SPINE

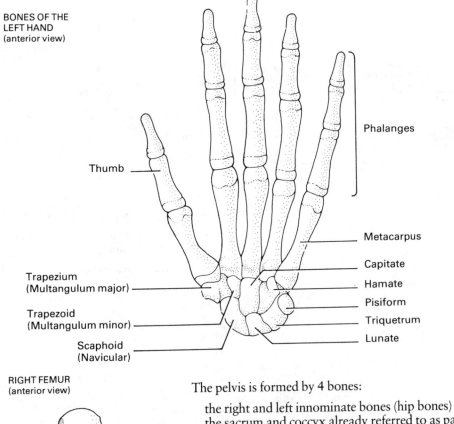

BONES OF THE
LEFT HAND
(anterior view)

Thumb

Phalanges

Metacarpus

Trapezium
(Multangulum major)

Capitate

Hamate

Trapezoid
(Multangulum minor)

Pisiform

Triquetrum

Scaphoid
(Navicular)

Lunate

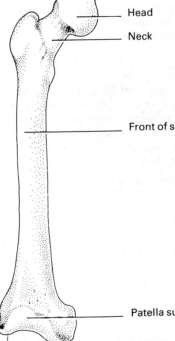

RIGHT FEMUR
(anterior view)

Head

Neck

Front of shaft

Patella surface

The pelvis is formed by 4 bones:

the right and left innominate bones (hip bones)
the sacrum and coccyx already referred to as part
of the spinal vertebrae.

Each innominate bone consists of:

the ilium—upper portion
the ischium—rear portion
the pubis—front portion.

60 bones go to form the lower limbs, 30 in each
whole leg:

the femur or thigh bone
the patella or kneecap
the tibia or shin bone
the fibula or brooch bone
7 tarsal bones of the ankle
5 metatarsal bones of the foot
14 phalanges of the toes.

BONES OF THE FOOT
(dorsal view)

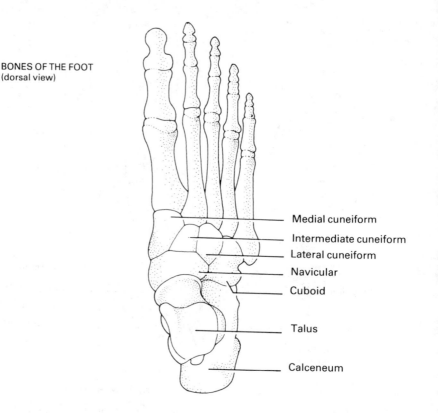

Medial cuneiform

Intermediate cuneiform

Lateral cuneiform

Navicular

Cuboid

Talus

Calceneum

In addition to the bones enumerated there is one hyoid bone which lies in the front upper part of the neck and is detached from the skeleton.

Spinal Curvature

Reference to the illustration of the spine shows that it has two natural curves—the slightly outward curving upper part of the spine being in the thoracic region and the inward curving of the spine being in the lumbar region. These natural curvatures can be exaggerated by three basic causes:

(1) *Congenital*—present at the time of birth or arising as a direct result of hereditary factors.

(2) *Traumatic*—resulting from accidents.

(3) *Environmental*—resulting from bad posture and often closely allied to the type of work in which the subject is engaged.

There are three types of curvature:

(1) Exaggerated outward curvature of the spine is referred to as *kyphosis*.

(2) An inward exaggeration of the spine is called *lordosis*.

(3) A lateral curvature of the spine is known as *scoliosis*. Scoliosis may occur at any part of the spine and is quite often associated with one of the other curvatures, e.g. the 'Hunchback of Notre Dame' suffered from kyphosis and scoliosis of the thoracic region.

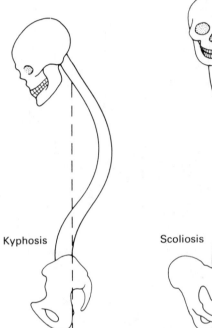
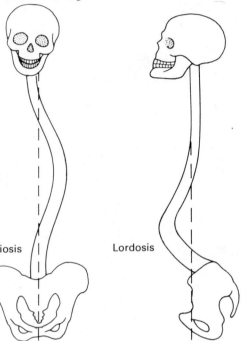

Kyphosis   Scoliosis   Lordosis

CURVATURE OF THE SPINE

Fractures

When a bone breaks it is referred to as a fracture; fractures are divided into a number of categories:

(1) *A simple fracture* is when a bone breaks in one place and no serious damage is done to the surrounding tissues.

(2) *A complicated fracture* is when the bone is broken and the break causes injury of the surrounding soft tissue.

(3) *A compound fracture* is when the bone is broken and one or both ends protrude through the external surface of the body, that is, through the skin.

(4) *A comminuted fracture* is where the bone is broken in a number of places.

(5) *An impacted fracture* is where the bone is broken and one end is driven into the other.

(6) *A greenstick fracture* is an incomplete fracture of a long bone as seen in young children.

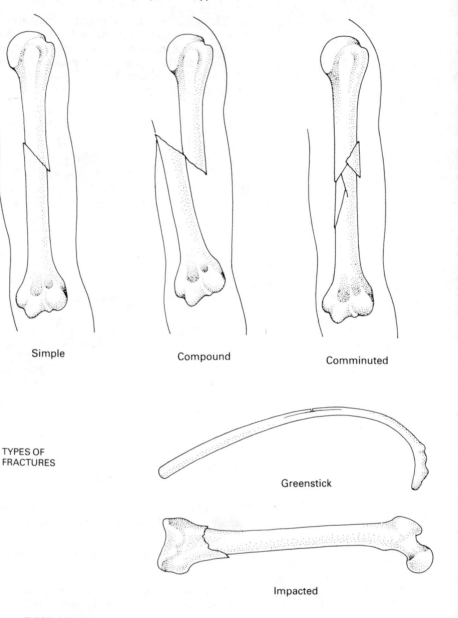

Simple

Compound

Comminuted

TYPES OF
FRACTURES

Greenstick

Impacted

DISEASES OF THE SKELETON

The skeleton is subject to many diseases, most of which do not come within the purview of this textbook, but mention must be made of arthritis because it is such a universal disease. Technically arthritis is an inflammation of a joint but this is generally interpreted as being a rheumatic affection of the joint, i.e. the inflammation is caused by the type of rheumatism which primarily affects the skeletal system as distinct from fibrositis and neuritis which are dealt with in later chapters.

There are many types of arthritis—among the more common being:

Mono-articular arthritis, as the name implies, is a type of arthritis which involves only one joint.

Poly-articular arthritis attacks a number of joints, usually associated joints, i.e. both hips or both knees or, in some cases, all the joints of one leg or arm.

Osteo- or degenerative arthritis is a chronic joint disease characterised by loss of some of the joint's cartilage and some spur formation.

Rheumatoid arthritis is a chronic arthritis usually associated with hormone deficiency.

Gouty arthritis (see glossary) is popularly associated with the big toe.

GLOSSARY

Appendicular Skeleton	skeleton of the upper and lower limbs and their girdles
Axial Skeleton	skeleton of the head and trunk
Cancellous Tissue	characterised by a latticed structure as seen in the spongy tissue of bones
Cartilage	a substance similar to bone but not as hard. It acts as a cushion between bones and also gives shape to nose and ears.
Dislocation	occurs when force is applied to a joint and is greater than that necessary to produce a strain. It particularly applies to the ball and socket joints as the ball is forced out of the socket. When dislocated bones are returned to their proper position this is referred to as *reduction.*
Gouty Arthritis	occurs in any part of the body but is popularly associated with the big toe. It results from urate crystals (chalky salts of uric acid) being deposited in and around the cartilage. This form of arthritis is much more common in men than women.
Orthopaedics	branch of surgery concerned with corrective treatment of skeletal system
Osteo	referring to bone
Periosteum	the hard membrane adhering to a bone and forming a protective cover. It contains blood vessels supplying blood to the bone and at its deepest layers are the bone-forming cells—osteoblasts.
Rickets	a calcium deficiency disease of children usually evidenced by misshapen bones.
Spondylitis	a type of arthritis which attacks the spinal vertebrae; the severest form is *ankylosing spondylitis* where bone and cartilage fuse resulting in complete immobility.

Chapter 3

The Muscular System

The main framework of the skeleton of the body is covered by muscles. These are responsible for 50 per cent of our body weight and their function is to permit movement, for which purpose they are, in most cases, attached to bones.

There are two types of muscle—*voluntary* and *involuntary*. The voluntary muscles, such as those used in walking or writing, are muscles which are under conscious control. Involuntary muscles are those which are involved in movements of the heart, respiration, digestion and so on, and are outside conscious control.

A section of *voluntary* muscle shows it to be of striped and striated (cross-banded) tissue whilst *involuntary* muscles have slender, smooth types of cells without cross stripes and are therefore usually referred to as smooth muscles.

A section of *cardiac* muscle tissue shows that whilst it is involuntary muscle it has characteristics which bear a superficial resemblance to voluntary muscle tissue though the fibres are smaller than those of voluntary muscles and the striae are not so well marked.

A muscle consists of a number of contractile or elastic fibres bound together in bundles. The bundles are, in turn, bound together by a thick band usually spindle-shaped and always contained in a sheath. This sheath is extended at the end to form strong fibrous bands known as the tendons by means of which the muscles are fastened to the bones.

CROSS-SECTION
THROUGH MUSCLE

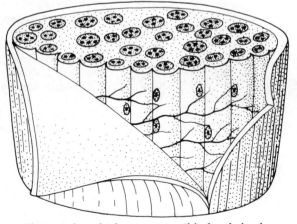

The muscles which are responsible for skeletal movements have two points of attachment—the point of origin is the bone to which they are attached and which they *do not* move and the point of insertion is the bone to which they are attached and which they *do* move, e.g. the biceps of the arm has its point of origin at the shoulder end of the arm, whilst the point of insertion is the radius of the lower arm—therefore it is the lower arm that is activated by the biceps.

A muscle receives its stimulus from a motor nerve and in response to this stimulus it shortens its lengh so that, *in action*, a muscle always contracts. Muscles in the body normally work in pairs. One is the prime mover and the other one holds it in check. This means that the muscles of the body—i.e. the voluntary muscles—are never completely at rest. They are normally in a condition of slight tension or contraction and this we call muscular tone.

By definition when one or more muscles are active in the initiation and maintenance of a movement they are called '*prime movers*' and when one or more muscles wholly oppose this they are referred to as '*antagonists*'. For example, when we bend our forearm the muscles on the front of the arm contract whilst, at the same time, the muscles on the back of the arm relax gradually to maintain balance. In this instance the muscles at the front of the arm are the prime movers whilst the ones at the back are the antagonists. However, to reverse this position and straighten the arm out again the muscles on the back of the arm become the prime movers and those on the front the antagonists.

Altogether there are some 640 named muscles in the body but there are many, many thousands of unnamed ones—each hair on the surface of the body having a tiny muscle attached to it. When a person gets chilled or frightened and has what are known as 'goose pimples'—the little lumps on the skin are due to the tiny muscles of the skin pulling the hair erect. Muscles are well supplied with arteries to bring them food for fuel and repair, and oxygen for combustion of the fuel, and with veins which carry away the waste products of their activities, such as carbon dioxide.

Muscular activity contributes materially to the internal heat of the body and when there is a danger of this reaching too low a level a person shivers. This is an involuntary action making the muscles work in order to generate more heat. Muscles are, in turn, responsive to exterior heat so that exposure of the skin to cold air increases muscle tone whereas considerable heat, e.g. a hot bath, has a relaxing effect on muscles. About 30 per cent of the energy produced in muscle activity results in work and the remaining 70 per cent is released as heat which warms the body, particularly the blood.

As previously mentioned in this chapter—muscle contraction occurs as the result of a stimulus which it receives from a motor nerve. This nerve stimulus sets up chemical changes in the muscles. These changes include the breaking down of glucose, glycogen and fat, which, in turn, liberate the energy required for contraction. In the process of contraction there are some waste products which are excreted from the muscles by the venous system. However, if at any one time the muscular activity is so great as to produce more waste products than the venous and lymph systems are able to cope with, then some waste products remain in the muscle or between the muscle fibres and give a feeling of stiffness—that is the fibres are no longer easily able to slide one over the other.

Muscles are put into groups according to the functions which they perform:

An extensor extends a limb.

A flexor flexes a limb.

An adductor bends a limb towards the median line.

An abductor takes a limb away from the median line.

A sphincter surrounds and closes an orifice or opening.

A supinator turns a limb to face upwards.

A pronator turns a limb to face downwards.

Rotators rotate a limb.

EXAMPLE OF
EXTENSOR MUSCLE

Triceps

EXAMPLE OF
FLEXOR MUSCLE

Biceps

The following is a short list of some of the principal muscles of the body. This is by no means a complete list and students who wish to study the subject in greater depth as well as to learn the origins and insertions of muscles are referred to one of the standard anatomical textbooks dealing with this subject. But this list should cover most, if not all, of the muscles that the physical therapist is likely to have to deal with.

Head and Neck

Name	Action
Epicraneas inc frontalis	elevates eyebrows and draws scalp forward
Orbicularis oculi	closes eyelids
Orbicularis oris	puckers mouth
Masseter	muscle of mastication, closes mouth, clenches teeth

MUSCLES OF THE BODY
(posterior view)

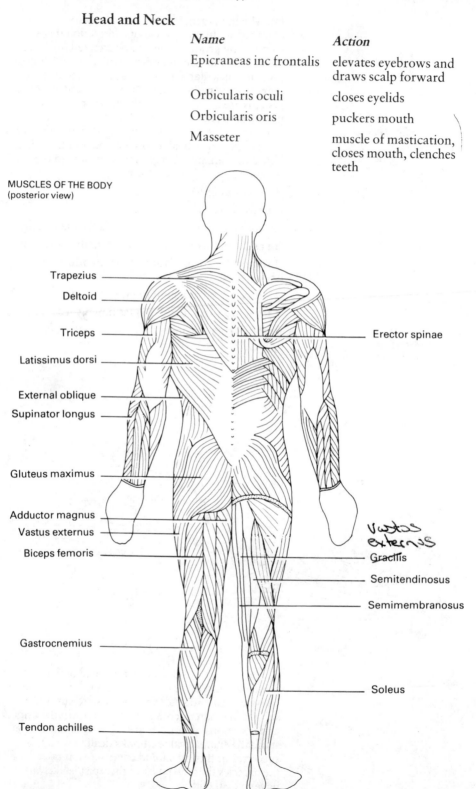

Trapezius

Deltoid

Triceps

Latissimus dorsi

External oblique

Supinator longus

Gluteus maximus

Adductor magnus

Vastus externus

Biceps femoris

Gastrocnemius

Tendon achilles

Erector spinae

Vastus externus

Gracilis

Semitendinosus

Semimembranosus

Soleus

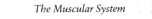

Name	Action
Buccinator	compresses cheeks and retracts angle of mouth
Sterno-cleido mastoid (Sterno-mastoid)	flexes head and turns from side to side
Platysma	muscle of facial expression

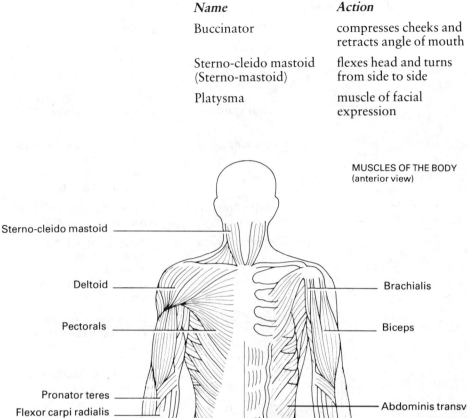

MUSCLES OF THE BODY
(anterior view)

Sterno-cleido mastoid

Deltoid

Pectorals

Pronator teres

Flexor carpi radialis

Flexor digitorum

Sartorius

Tibialis anterior

Brachialis

Biceps

Abdominis transversalis

External oblique

Abdominis rectus

Vastus externus (lateralis)

Gracilis

Adductor magnus

Vastus internus (medialis)

Trunk of Body

Name	*Action*
Trapezius	rotates inferior angle of scapula laterally, raises shoulder, draws scapula backwards
Erector spinae	extends vertebral column
Latissimus dorsi	adducts the shoulder and draws the arm backwards and downwards
Serratus anterior (serratus magnus)	draws the scapula forward
Gluteus maximus	extends hip joint and extends trunk on buttocks in raising body from sitting position
Psoas	flexes hip joint and trunk on lower extremities

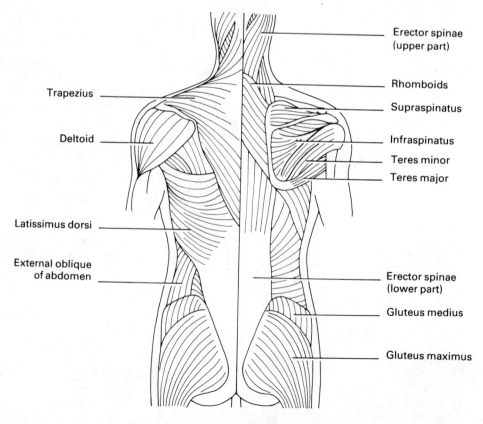

MUSCLES OF THE BACK

Name	Action
Pectoralis major	Flexes shoulder joint, depresses shoulder girdle, adducts and rotates humerus
Abdominis obliquus (internal and external oblique)	supports abdominal viscera and flexes vertebral column
Abdominis transversalis (transversus abdominis)	supports abdominal viscera and flexes vertebral column
Abdominis rectus	supports abdominal viscera and flexes vertebral column

The Arms

Name	Action
Deltoid	abduction of the humerus to right angle
Biceps brachialis	flexes and supinates forearm
Triceps brachialis	extends elbow joint
Brachialis	flexes elbow joint
Coraco brachialis	flexes and adducts humerus
Brachioradialis (supinator longus)	flexes elbow joint
Pronator teres (pronator radii teres)	pronates forearm
Supinator (supinator radii brevis)	supinates forearm
Flexor carpi radialis	flexes wrist joint
Extensor carpi (radialis longus)	extends wrist
Flexor carpi ulnaris	flexes wrist joint
Extensor carpi ulnaris	extends wrist joint
Flexor digitorum	flexes fingers
Extensor digitorum	extends fingers

The Legs

Name	Action
Rectus femoris (Quadriceps)	extends knee joint
Vastus lateralis (externus) (Quadriceps)	extends knee joint
Vastus medialis (internus) (Quadriceps)	extends knee joint
Vastus intermedius (Quadriceps)	extends knee joint
Sartorius	flexes hip and knee joints and rotates femur
Adductor magnus, longus, and brevis	adducts thigh
Biceps femoris	flexes knee joint

Name	Action
Semitendinosus (ham string)	flexes knee joint and extends hip joint
Semimembranosus (ham string)	flexes knee joint and extends hip joint
Gracilis	adducts femur and flexes knee joint
Gastrocnemius	flexes ankle and knee joint
Tibialis anterior (tibialis anticus)	extends and inverts foot
Peroneus longus	everts and flexes foot and supports arches
Flexor digitorum longus	flexes toes
Extensor digitorum longus	extends toes
Tendon of achilles	assists in flexion of the foot
Soleus	flexes ankle joint
Sartorius	flexes hip and knee joints and rotates femur laterally

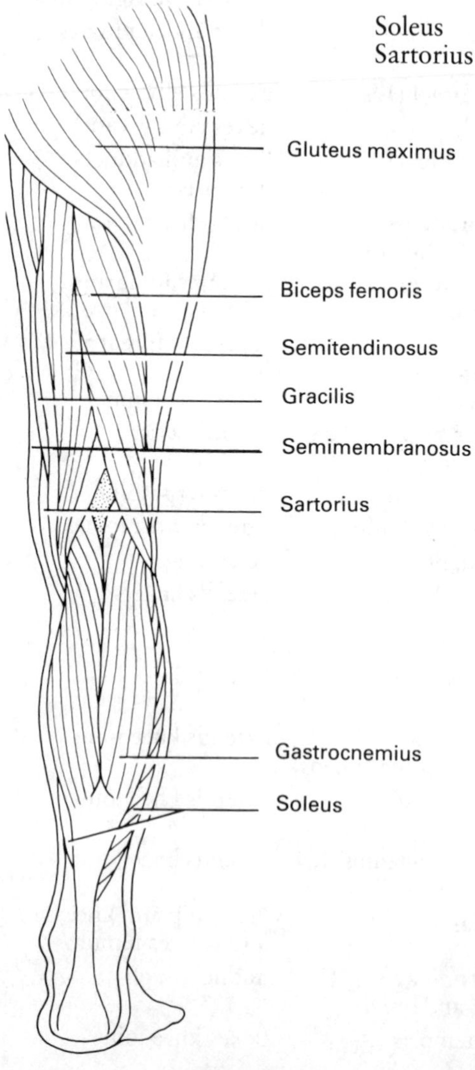

Gluteus maximus

Biceps femoris

Semitendinosus

Gracilis

Semimembranosus

Sartorius

Gastrocnemius

Soleus

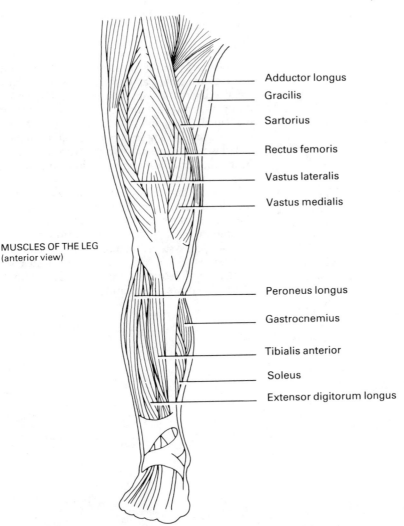

Adductor longus

Gracilis

Sartorius

Rectus femoris

Vastus lateralis

Vastus medialis

MUSCLES OF THE LEG
(anterior view)

Peroneus longus

Gastrocnemius

Tibialis anterior

Soleus

Extensor digitorum longus

COMMON DISEASES OR CONDITIONS AFFECTING THE MUSCULAR SYSTEM

One of the most common diseases of the system is *fibrositis* which technically means inflammation of soft tissue and is a term which is now generally applied to a rheumatic affection of the muscles—a condition in which there is a build-up of urea and lactic acid inside the muscle to the extent of causing stiffness and pain.

A well known example of this disease is *lumbago* or fibrositis of muscles in the lumbar region. *Torticollis* or 'wry neck' is another condition which has much in common with muscular fibrositis. In this case the muscle concerned is the sterno-cleido mastoid muscle of the neck which, in a state of contraction, causes the head to take up an abnormal position.

Another common condition is that of *cramp*. This is a localised painful contraction of one or more muscles, which has a number of causes, the most usual being that of vigorous exercise; but it also occurs in certain metabolic disorders, e.g. when there is a sodium depletion or water depletion. It is for the purpose of avoiding cramp that copious quantities of salted water are given to people who work in intense heat – for example, people who look after furnaces at steelworks.

There are also disease conditions which affect muscles though their cause is to be found in one of the other systems. For example, *poliomyelitis*—commonly called 'polio'—which arises in the neurological system and multiple or disseminated *sclerosis* which also arises in the neurological system, though both these disease conditions profoundly affect the body's musculature.

GLOSSARY

Atony	abnormally low degree of tonus or absence of it
Atrophy	reduction in the size of a muscle which previously reached a matured size; popularly referred to as wastage
Cramp	painful involuntary contraction of muscle
Fascia	the sheath or membrane covering a muscle
Ganglion	a cystic swelling which occurs in association with a joint or tendon sheath. Ganglia most commonly occur on the back of the wrist
Myology	the science of muscles
Myositis	inflammation of a muscle
Ligaments	bands of fibrous tissue which help to bind the bones of joints together
Rupture	a tearing or bursting of the fascia or sheath which surrounds the fibres of the muscle
Spasm	a sudden muscular contraction
Sprain	an injury to a ligament
Strain	an injury to a muscle or its tendon
Tendon	a band of fibrous tissue forming the end of a muscle and attaching it to the bone
Tonus	muscle tone
Viscera	the contents of the abdominal cavity

Chapter 4   The Vascular System

This system, which is sometimes called the circulatory system, consists of the heart, blood vessels, blood, lymphatic vessels and lymph.

The centre of this system is the heart, which is a muscular organ that rhythmically contracts, forcing the blood through a system of vessels. The heart weighs approximately 255 g in a fully grown adult and lies one-third to the right and two-thirds to the left of the thoracic cavity. At birth it beats about 130 times a minute, at six years about 100 times a minute, reducing in adult life to between 65 and 80 beats a minute with an average somewhere around 70. During the 24 hour period an adult human heart pumps 36 000 litres of blood through the 20 000 km of blood vessels.

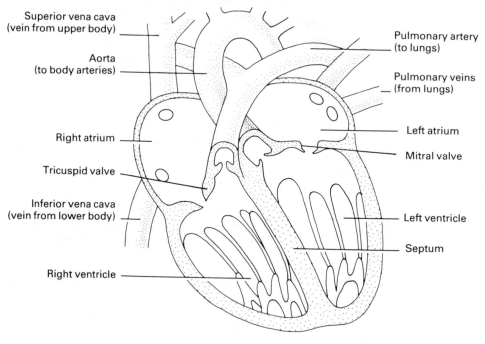

Superior vena cava (vein from upper body)

Aorta (to body arteries)

Right atrium

Tricuspid valve

Inferior vena cava (vein from lower body)

Right ventricle

Pulmonary artery (to lungs)

Pulmonary veins (from lungs)

Left atrium

Mitral valve

Left ventricle

Septum

THE HEART

The heart is divided into four chambers. These are the right and the left *atria (or auricles)*, in the upper part of the heart, and the right and left *ventricles* in the lower part. The right side of the heart is divided from the left by a solid wall or *septum* which prevents the venous blood on the right side coming into contact with the arterial blood on the left side of the heart.

Circulation is divided into two principal systems: the *general* or *systemic* circulation (around the body); and the *pulmonary* circulation (to and from the lungs).

The general circulation includes two special branches: the *portal* circulation, which conveys blood from the digestive organs to the liver; and the *coronary* circulation, which supplies the heart.

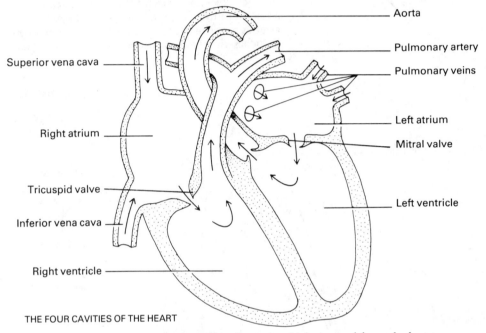

Aorta

Pulmonary artery

Pulmonary veins

Superior vena cava

Left atrium

Right atrium

Mitral valve

Tricuspid valve

Left ventricle

Inferior vena cava

Right ventricle

THE FOUR CAVITIES OF THE HEART

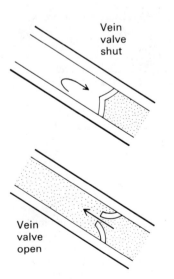

Vein valve shut

Vein valve open

VEINS
(convey blood to the heart)

Blood vessels which proceed from the heart are known as *arteries*. They generally carry oxygenated blood (the exception being the pulmonary artery). They are large, hollow, elastic tubes which gradually decrease in diameter as they spread through the body. These smaller vessels or *arteries* finally become very fine hairlike vessels known as *capillaries*.

Blood vessels which proceed towards the heart are known as veins. They generally carry deoxygenated blood (the exception being the pulmonary vein). They are elastic tubes with valves which prevent a backward flow of blood.

The veins empty the deoxygenated blood into the right atrium of the heart from the *inferior* and *superior vena cava*. The blood flows through the *tricuspid* valve to the right ventricle and is pumped to the lungs via the pulmonary artery. This is the only artery in the body to carry deoxygenated blood.

The blood is reoxygenated in the lungs and returns to the left atrium of the heart through the pulmonary veins. These are the only veins to transport oxygenated blood. The blood flows into the left ventricle through the *mitral* valve and is pumped to the body through the *aorta*.

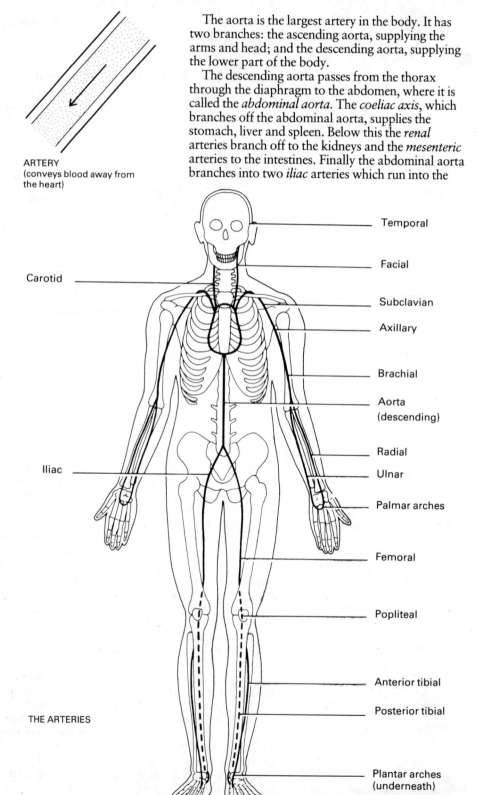

The aorta is the largest artery in the body. It has two branches: the ascending aorta, supplying the arms and head; and the descending aorta, supplying the lower part of the body.

The descending aorta passes from the thorax through the diaphragm to the abdomen, where it is called the *abdominal aorta*. The *coeliac axis*, which branches off the abdominal aorta, supplies the stomach, liver and spleen. Below this the *renal* arteries branch off to the kidneys and the *mesenteric* arteries to the intestines. Finally the abdominal aorta branches into two *iliac* arteries which run into the

ARTERY
(conveys blood away from
the heart)

Temporal

Facial

Carotid

Subclavian

Axillary

Brachial

Aorta
(descending)

Radial

Ulnar

Iliac

Palmar arches

Femoral

Popliteal

Anterior tibial

Posterior tibial

THE ARTERIES

Plantar arches
(underneath)

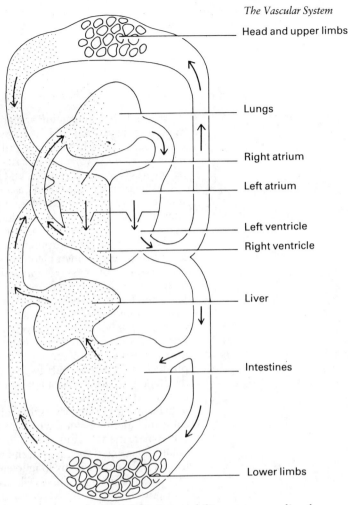

Head and upper limbs

Lungs

Right atrium

Left atrium

Left ventricle

Right ventricle

Liver

Intestines

Lower limbs

DIRECTION OF
CIRCULATION

pelvis. The *internal iliac* artery supplies the
reproductive organs while the *external iliac* artery
becomes the *femoral* artery which is the main artery
of the lower limb.

The femoral artery supplies the thigh muscles and
becomes the *popliteal* artery at the knee. This divides
into the *anterior* and *posterior tibial* arteries. The
anterior tibial artery supplies the front of the leg and
is continued to the foot as the *dorsalis pedis* artery.
The posterior tibial artery supplies the back of the leg
and reaches the sole of the foot as the *plantar artery*
which forms the *plantar arches*.

Two *coronary* arteries branch off the ascending
aorta, which then passes upwards as the *innominate*
artery. This divides into the *subclavian* and *carotid*
arteries.

The subclavian artery passes behind the clavicle
and enters the armpit where it becomes the *axillary*
artery. The *brachial* artery continues for the length of
the upper arm until the elbow where it divides into
the *radial* and *ulnar* arteries, culminating in the
palmar arches in the hand.

The carotid artery passes upwards to the neck and has four main branches, the *facial, temporal, occipital* and maxillary arteries.

BLOOD

Blood is alkaline in reaction and amounts to approximately 5–6 litres in the average adult. It is complex in nature but has four principal constituent parts—*plasma, erythrocytes* or red corpuscles, *leucocytes* or white corpuscles and *platelets.*

Plasma provides the liquid basis of the blood. This is a clear, straw-coloured liquid which holds various substances in solution. These include sugar, urea, amino acids, mineral salts, enzymes, etc.

Erythrocytes or red corpuscles (corpuscles is Latin for little bodies) are inert biconcave discs, they get their colour from haemoglobin which has the ability to absorb oxygen (when it becomes *oxy-haemoglobin* which is bright red in colour) and carbon dioxide (when it becomes *carboxy-haemoglobin* which becomes very dark red, bordering on a muddy brown colour). The average life span of an erythrocyte is 120 days; they are produced in red bone marrow and their eventual disintegration takes place in the spleen, and is finally completed in the liver.

In health, the erythrocytes total about 5 million per cubic millimetre of blood which gives a total of somewhere in the region of 25 billion in a human adult. If these cells were placed end to end they would form a ribbon sufficiently long to encircle the world more than four times. These cells are the body's transporters; they carry oxygen to all parts of the body and on their return journey pick up waste products, primarily carbon dioxide.

Leucocytes or phagocytes (white corpuscles) are larger than erythrocytes and have an irregular shape and a nucleus. They are produced in the bone marrow and, in health, they total about 8000 per cubic millimetre. They are the protectors or soldiers of the body; their chief role is to protect the body against infection by their power of ingesting bacteria—a process which is known as *phagocytosis.* When the body is subject to serious infection the leucocytes increase rapidly by a process of division known as mitosis.

Then we have platelets or thrombocytes. These average 250 000 per cubic millimetre of blood. They are derived from large multinucleated cells in the bone marrow and are essential to the blood for coagulation, i.e. clotting.

Blood Types

The existence of human blood types was established by Karl Landsteiner in 1902 when he began a study to determine why fatalities occurred following some blood transfusions. He discovered that the cause was incompatibility between the blood of the donor and the blood of the recipient.

Arising from this work came the Landsteiner Classification of Blood Groups which classified blood into the four types A, B, AB and O.

Type O is called the universal donor because it may give blood to all blood types but it can only receive from type O. On the other hand, type AB is called the universal recipient because it can receive from any group but can only give to the AB group. Type A can give to both A and AB and receive only from types A and O. Type B can give to type B and AB and receive only from types B or O.

In 1940 Landsteiner and A. S. Weiner recognised the Rh factor, a substance found in red blood cells.

LYMPH NODES

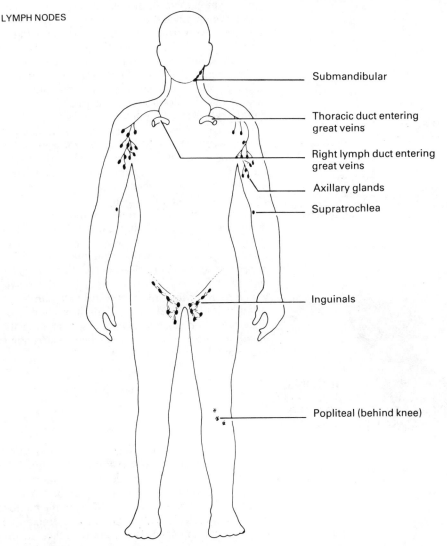

Submandibular

Thoracic duct entering great veins

Right lymph duct entering great veins

Axillary glands

Supratrochlea

Inguinals

Popliteal (behind knee)

This was discovered during their experiments with rhesus monkeys, hence the name rhesus or the abbreviation Rh. It is estimated that 85 per cent of white people have Rh positive factor and the other 15 per cent are Rh negative.

THE LYMPHATIC SYSTEM

This is a secondary circulation intertwined with the blood circulation. The basic material of the lymphatic system is the *lymph* which is plasma after it has been exuded from the capillaries. It gives nourishment to the tissue cells and in return takes away their waste products. The liquid is drained off by tiny lymphatic vessels which join together to form larger lymph vessels and, as these lymph vessels convey lymph towards the heart, they are supplied with valves in much the same way as veins. Along their course towards the heart there are receiving or reservoir areas known as *lymph nodes*. They vary in size from a pin head to a small almond. The purpose of these lymph nodes is to filter the lymph as it passes through and, in this way, to help prevent infection passing into the blood stream and to add *lymphocytes* to the lymph.

Eventually all lymph passes into two principal lymph vessels, the *thoracic duct* and the right *lymphatic duct*, which open into the blood stream at the junctions of the right and left internal, jugular and subclavian veins where it becomes part of the general systemic circulation again.

There are approximately 100 of these lymphatic nodes scattered throughout the body along the line of the lymphatic vessels. The most common superficial ones are the *inguinals* in the groin, the nodes in the *popliteal fossa* or depression behind the knee, the *supratrochlea* in the crutch of the elbow, the *axillary glands* in the armpit, the *supraclavicular glands*, the *submandibular glands* underneath the mandible and the *cervical* and *occipital glands*. These superficial glands are the ones which swell when an infection is present in that part of the body.

CONDITIONS, DEFICIENCIES AND DISEASES OF THE VASCULAR SYSTEM

Probably the most common blood complaint is that of *anaemia* which means loss of normal balance between the productive and destructive blood processes. This can be due to a drop in the blood volume after a haemorrage, or a drop in the number of red blood cells, or in the amount of haemoglobin, or a combination of any two or more of these factors.

There are many forms of anaemia but we are primarily concerned with two categories, *simple anaemia* and *pernicious anaemia*.

In simple anaemia there are two direct causative factors, the first is a marked nutritional deficiency of iron, frequently seen in the premature infant, the growing child, and the pregnant woman. The second causative factor is chronic blood loss, for example during menstruation or because of accident.

One of the characteristics of pernicious anaemia is the presence of giant red cells (*macrocytes*), each cell appearing to be overloaded with haemoglobin, whilst the total red cells count is decreased. As recently as 1925 this disease was invariably fatal— today the life expectancy of the properly treated patient is about the same as that of the general population. Basically, pernicious anaemia results from failure of red blood cells to develop and mature normally.

Whilst a decreased number of red blood cells is indicative of anaemia a continously increasing number of white blood cells can be indicative of *leukaemia*. Reference has already been made to the fact that white blood cells increase in number by mitosis in the presence of the necessary stimuli such as an infection and the normal 8000 per cubic millimetre of blood can increase to as many as 60 000 in a case of severe pneumonia. However, when the condition is cured, the mitosing or dividing ceases and the white blood count returns to normal. In leukaemia the leucocytes and/or lymphocytes do not remain at the normal number but gradually increase.

Varicose Veins

A network of veins serves to drain the capillary beds and body tissue of 'used' blood, and returns this blood to the heart. Venous flow is assisted in its return to the heart by the rhythmic suction action of breathing, muscular contraction in the extremities and the valves located in the veins. Gravity assists the venous blood from the neck and head to return to the heart but venous flow from the legs is against the pull of gravity and, for most of the day, has to run uphill. The valves in the veins prevent back flow and when some of these valves become impaired or cease to function the veins become permanently dilated. There are many causes of varicosity but these include:

(1) *Congenital factors*: varicosity appears to run in families.
(2) *Environmental factors*: people whose work necessitates their standing still for long periods of time are at particular risk.

Varicose veins are also, quite often, a complication of pregnancy and obesity.

Haemophilia

This is the best known of the bleeding diseases. It is a hereditary disease—the victim is always male and the disease is passed on by the mother, who is the so-called carrier. It is a disease in which there is a deficiency in the clotting of the blood.

Blue Baby

This is a baby born with a congenital structural defect of the heart which results in a constant recirculation of some of the venous blood without its prior passage through the lungs to pick up oxygen. The degree of blueness is, at least in part, dependent on the size of the hole through which the venous blood passes.

Arteriosclerosis and Atherosclerosis

These two conditions are often confused because of the similarity in many of the symptoms.

Simply, arteriosclerosis is hardening of the arterial walls brought about mainly by degenerative changes which increase in frequency with age. In atherosclerosis—there is a build up of cholesterol on the inside of the artery which reduces the size of the bore.

BLOOD TRANSFUSIONS

The transfer of blood to a recipient from a donor is one of the very widely used procedures in medical treatments—making up deficiencies caused by severe haemorrhage and, in some cases, when the blood volume is normal, a transfusion is used in order to replace a deficiency in one of the constituents of the blood.

The first record we have of a transfusion was of one performed between two dogs by a Richard Lower in England in 1665. Soon after this it was tried in France but the results on humans were so disastrous that the French passed a law forbidding transfusions. It was not until the early 20th century, when Karl Landsteiner completed his blood grouping, that progress was made in the field of human transfusions. Because, at that time, they had no means of keeping the blood fresh—only direct transfusions were possible. In 1914 Louis Agote of Argentina found that sodium citrate could be used for this purpose and the discovery was used extensively in the First World War. Since that time new methods have been found for obtaining and keeping blood for use at some future time and blood banks have become an accepted part of our medical system.

GLOSSARY

Angiology	the science dealing with blood vessels and lymphatics
Cholesterol	a constituent of all animal fats and oils, insoluble in water. Its presence on the inside walls of blood vessels contributes to hypertension and other cardio-vascular conditions
Coronary	relating to the blood (heart area)
Diastolic Pressure	the pressure measured during the relaxing phase of the cardiac cycle
Electrocardiogram (ECG)	a graphic record of heart activity made on an instrument known as an electro-cardiograph
Haemorrhoids (Piles)	dilated veins in the rectum and anus, described as internal or external depending on their position
Hypertension	high blood pressure
Hypotension	low blood pressure
Phlebitis	an inflammation of the vein walls, most common in the legs. It may lead to thrombo-phlebitis, a complication caused by an obstructing blood clot.
Systolic Pressure	the pressure measured during the contraction phase of the cardiac cycle
Thrombus	a clot of blood found within the heart or blood vessels
Tricuspid and *Mitral*	valves of the heart

Chapter 5

The Neurological System

The neurological system of the body has two main divisions—

(1) **The central** (or cerebrospinal) *nervous system*.
(2) **The autonomic** (including the sympathetic and parasympathetic) *nervous system*.

The basis of the nervous system is the *nerve cell* or *neuron*. This consists of a nerve cell body with its receiving processes—the *dendrites*, its transmitting process—the *axon* and its *nerve endings*. White nerve fibres are *medullated*, that is they are enclosed in a sheath of *myelin*. Grey nerve fibres are non-medullated, that is, they have no myelin.

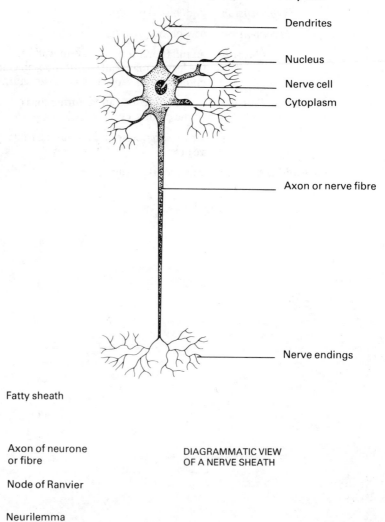

A NEURON

Dendrites

Nucleus

Nerve cell

Cytoplasm

Axon or nerve fibre

Nerve endings

Fatty sheath

Axon of neurone or fibre

Node of Ranvier

Neurilemma

DIAGRAMMATIC VIEW
OF A NERVE SHEATH

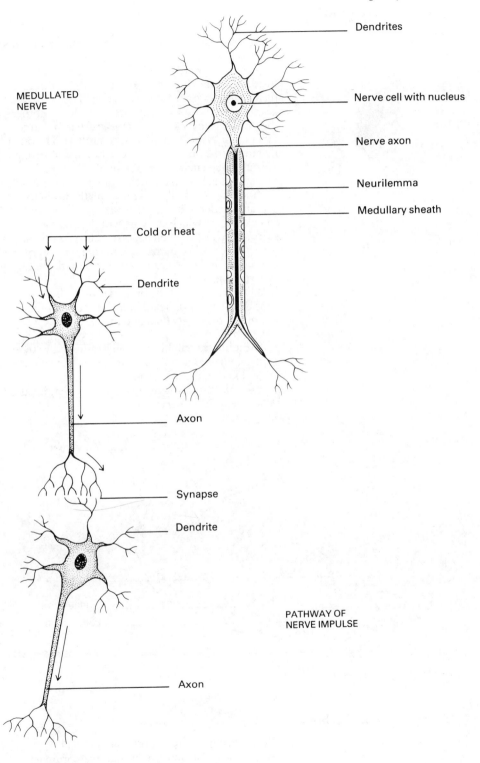

MEDULLATED
NERVE

Dendrites

Nerve cell with nucleus

Nerve axon

Neurilemma

Medullary sheath

Cold or heat

Dendrite

Axon

Synapse

Dendrite

PATHWAY OF
NERVE IMPULSE

Axon

THE BRAIN

At the centre of the nervous system is the brain. This, as has already been seen, is well protected from the outside by the hard bone structure of the skull. Inside, the brain is protected externally by three membranes known as the *meninges*. The outer layer is known as the *dura mater* (strong or hard mother), the middle layer is known as the *arachnoid* and the inner layer as the *pia mater* (soft mother). The outer meninges (the dura mater) is constructed of strong fibrous tissue anchored to the skull. The middle tissue, or arachnoid, is much more delicate and is not anchored to the skull, thus allowing the brain to expand. Under it lies the big reservoir of cerebral spinal fluid by which the whole of the brain is surrounded and on which it rests. Then comes the pia mater which is in contact with the grey matter of the brain itself and dips deep down between the brain convolutions.

When we speak of the brain we are really considering three quite different structures—the *cerebrum*, the *cerebellum* and the *medulla oblongata*.

The adult human brain weighs rather more than 1360 g and is so full of water that it tends to slump rather like a blancmange if placed without the support of a firm surface. It is estimated that it has 12 billion neurons or nerve cells.

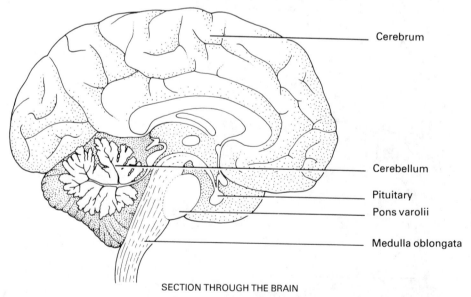

SECTION THROUGH THE BRAIN

The Cerebrum

The cerebrum consists of two symmetrical hemispheres. The outer layer of the cerebrum is known as the *cortex* and this is arranged in convolutions, that is, deep irregularly shaped fissures or indentations. This is the grey matter of the brain. Underneath the cortex lies nerve fibre or white matter. The function of the cerebrum is to control voluntary movement and to receive and interpret conscious sensations. It is the seat of the higher functions such as the senses, memory, reasoning, intelligence and moral sense.

The Cerebellum

The cerebellum is much smaller in size and lies below and behind the cerebrum. It too has grey matter under which is white matter. Its function is to control muscular co-ordination and balance.

The Medulla Oblongata

The medulla oblongata is about 3 cm long, tapering from its greatest width of 2 cm and connecting the rest of the brain with the spinal cord with which it is continuous. It is made up of interspersed white and grey matter. The medulla oblongata not only acts as the link between the brain and the central nervous system of the body but it is also the centre of those parts of the autonomic nervous system which control the heart, lungs, processes of digestion, etc.

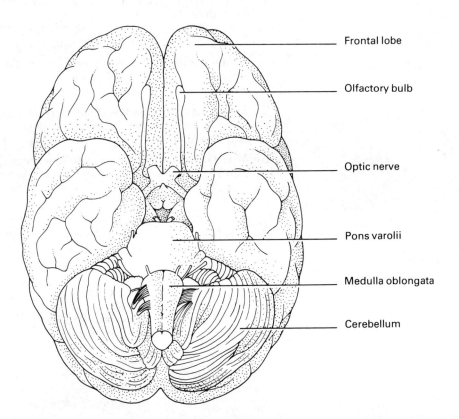

Frontal lobe

Olfactory bulb

Optic nerve

Pons varolii

Medulla oblongata

Cerebellum

The Spinal Cord

The spinal cord, which is continuous with the medulla oblongata, extends downwards through the vertebrae of the spinal column. The cord itself is cylindrical in shape with an outer covering of supporting cells and blood vessels and an inner egg-shaped core of nerve fibres. It extends through four-fifths of the spinal column and is about 45 cm in length.

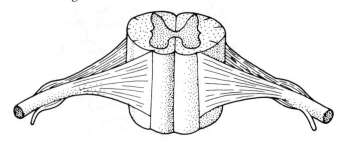

There are 12 pairs of cranial nerves given off from the base of the brain; 31 other pairs branch off the spinal cord throughout its length. These extend to every part of the body. Nerves that extend upwards through the spinal cord to the brain pass through the medulla oblongata where they cross – thus the left-hand side of the brain controls the right-hand side of the body whilst the right-hand side of the brain controls the left-hand side of the body. Nerves of the central nervous system fall into three categories.

(1) *Motor or efferent nerves*—the primary function of these nerves is to control the movement of muscles.

(2) *Sensory or afferent nerves*—these carry impulses from the sensory nerve endings to the spinal column and the brain.

(3) *Mixed nerves*—these consist of both motor and sensory fibres.

Cranial Nerves

Name	Type	Function	No.
abducent	motor	supplies lateral rectus muscles of eyes	VI
auditory	sensory	sense of hearing, maintenance of balance, equilibrium	VIII
facial	mixed	sense of taste from tongue and impulses to muscles of facial expression	VII
glosso-pharyngeal	mixed	sensations from tongue, impulses to muscles of pharynx	IX

Name	Type	Function	No.
hypoglossal	motor	supplies tongue muscles	XII
oculomotor	motor	supplies muscles operating eyes	III
olfactory	sensory	sense of smell	I
optic	sensory	sense of sight	II
trochlear	motor	supplies superior oblique muscles of eyes	IV
trigeminal	mixed	receiving pain, heat, pressure and stimulating muscles of mastication	V
spinal accessory	motor	to sterno-cleido mastoid and trapezius muscles	XI
vagus	mixed	sensory, motor, digestive and respiratory organs	X

The 31 pairs of spinal nerves comprise 8 pairs of *cervical nerves*, 12 pairs of *thoracic nerves*, 5 pairs of *lumbar nerves*, 5 pairs of *sacral nerves* and 1 pair of *coccygeal nerves*.

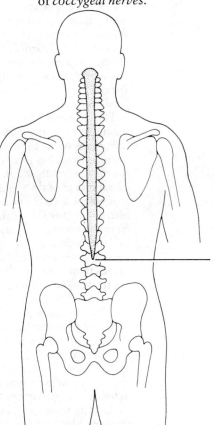

POSITION OF
SPINAL CORD

Cord ends between
1st and 2nd
lumbar vetebrae

Other parts of the brain include the *pons varolii* which is a bridge of nerve fibres linking the right and left hemispheres and also the cerebellum with the cerebrum above and the medulla oblongata below. All impulses which pass between the brain and the spinal cord traverse the pons varolii.

The Pituitary Gland (or Hypophysis)

The pituitary gland (or hypophysis) is a small gland about the size of a pea and lies in the pituitary fossa in the base of the skull. Its function is dealt with in the chapter on the endocrine system.

The Hypothalamus

The hypothalamus is situated in the area of the floor of the third ventricle of the brain and it exercises an influence over the autonomic nervous system. It contains the heat regulating centre and is generally believed to be involved with appetite.

THE AUTONOMIC NERVOUS SYSTEM

This supplies all body structures over which we have no voluntary control. It is divided into two separate parts—the *sympathetic system* and the *parasympathetic system*.

The sympathetic system comprises a gangliated cord which runs on either side of the front of the vertebral column. The principal plexuses of this system are: the *cardiac plexus* which supplies all the thoracic viscera and the thoracic vessels; the *coeliac* or *solar plexus* which supplies all the abdominal viscera and the *hypogastric plexus* which supplies the pelvic organs.

The parasympathetic nervous system consists mainly of the vagus nerve which gives off branches to the organs of the thorax and abdomen, but also includes branches from other cranial nerves, mainly the third, seventh and ninth as well as nerves in the sacral region of the spinal column.

It will be seen from the above notes that all the internal organs therefore have a double nerve supply from the sympathetic and parasympathetic systems and their effect is opposite—simply, a sympathetic nerve has the effect of increasing body activity and speeds it up, whereas the parasympathetic, on the contrary, slows down body activity.

The sympathetic fibres increase the heart rate, raise the blood pressure, mobilise glucose, stimulate the secretion of sweat. The parasympathetic fibres slow the heart, lower the blood pressure and decrease the secretion of sweat. It has been maintained that the sympathetic system provides for today's work and that its action increases when involved with physical activity. The parasympathetic—on the other hand—looks after tomorrow, being mainly concerned with changes which take place during rest.

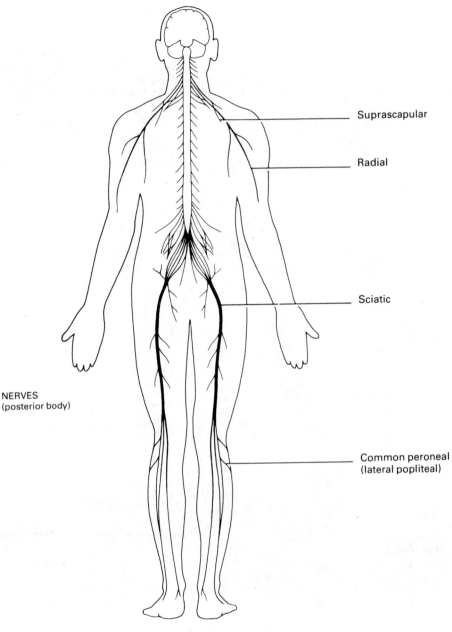

Suprascapular

Radial

Sciatic

Common peroneal
(lateral popliteal)

NERVES
(posterior body)

The sympathetic nerves are stimulated by strong emotions such as anger and excitement. In fact it is because of this effect of the emotions that they are called sympathetic.

The *adrenal* is one of the glands which they stimulate and the liberation of *adrenalin* is one of the body's responses to anger. In some people, the parasympathetic nerves are the stronger and hold the balance in the body; such people generally have a placid disposition, good digestion and are not very easily disturbed. These are known as *vagotonic types*. In other people, the sympathetic nerves are the stronger and these people are more emotional, less stable and their digestion is more readily disturbed. These are known as *sympatheticotonic types*.

Another function of the autonomic nervous system is related to the reflex nervous action. This is an involuntary reaction to a stimulation, for

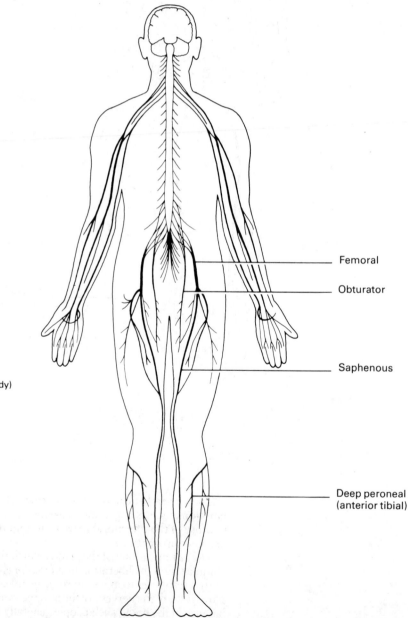

NERVES
(anterior body)

Femoral

Obturator

Saphenous

Deep peroneal
(anterior tibial)

example, taking the fingers away quickly from a hot surface, the recovery of balance to prevent a fall, and so on. It is also within this system that a reflex action is *conditioned*. For example, the normal reflex action when handed a very hot plate would be to drop it, but as this action would carry with it certain distinct disadvantages, like loss of the meal that was on the plate or the work involved with clearing up afterwards, the plate—instead of being dropped—is quickly put down. That is a reflex action which has been conditioned by other considerations.

CONDITIONS AND DISEASES OF THE NEUROLOGICAL SYSTEM

Neuritis

This takes in a wide group of disturbances which affect the peripheral nerves after they leave the spinal cord. Some of the disturbances are due to infection—others to compression of the nerves. Probably the biggest single factor is the build-up of urea and lactic acid at a point, or points, of the nerve's course, which affects the nerve's sheathing.

Bell's Palsy or Facial Paralysis

A neuritis of the facial nerve usually caused by infection and compression of the swollen nerve as it passes through a tiny opening in the skull below the ear in its course to the muscles of the face.

Neuralgia

This is a painful condition in a nerve due to irritation, inflammation or exposure.

Parkinson's Disease

Otherwise known as Paralysis Agitans, this is an extremely common illness beginning in middle life, deriving from disease of the basal ganglia. The disease is slowly progressive but as it does not affect the brain there is no loss of speech and intelligence is unaffected. The chief symptoms of this illness are tremor, rigidity and slowness of movement.

Sciatica

This is inflammation of the great sciatic nerve, the longest single nerve in the body. This is often a form of rheumatic neuritis but it can also be caused by compression, an arthritic spur or a slipped disc.

GLOSSARY

Brachial Neuritis   a condition similar to sciatica but in the arm

Ganglion   a group of nerve cell bodies usually located outside the brain and spinal cord

Plexus   a network of interlacing nerves

Spasticity   a stage of sustained contraction of a muscle associated with an exaggeration of deep reflexes

Synapse   the region of communication between neurons; the point at which an impulse passes from an axon of one neuron to a dendrite of the cell body of another

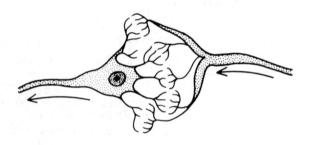

NERVE SYNAPSE

Chapter 6

The Digestive System

This is the system which is responsible for changing the food, which is *put into* the body, into substances suitable for absorption and therefore *usable by* the body. As the health and efficient working of the body must depend, to a very large extent, on the food which is put into it and the treatment which the food receives—it is necessary to have at least a basic understanding of the processes involved and some of

THE DIGESTIVE
SYSTEM

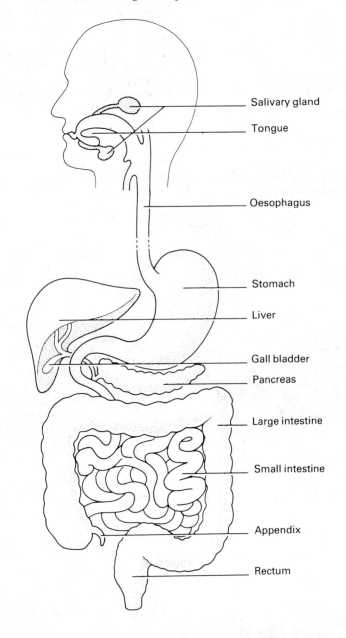

Salivary gland

Tongue

Oesophagus

Stomach

Liver

Gall bladder

Pancreas

Large intestine

Small intestine

Appendix

Rectum

the ways in which they may go wrong. The body needs material for growth, repair, heat and energy and these materials are supplied by the foods we eat. It is the digestive system which produces the chemical and other changes which make it possible for the food to perform functions necessary to maintain life.

Digestive juices contain *enzymes* which break down food. Enzymes are proteins which speed up chemical reactions; they are biological *catalysts*.

The digestive tract or alimentary canal is more than 10 m long. It is continuous, starting at the mouth, passing through the pharynx, the oesophagus, the stomach, the small and large intestine and ending with the rectum and the anus. Associated with it are accessory organs: the *tongue, teeth, salivary glands, liver* and *pancreas.* Starting with the teeth—there are 32 permanent teeth; working from the front backwards on each side of the jaw, there are *two incisors, one canine* or eye tooth, *two premolars* or bicuspids and *three molars.*

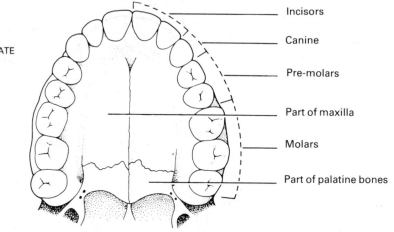

THE TEETH
AND BONY PALATE

Incisors

Canine

Pre-molars

Part of maxilla

Molars

Part of palatine bones

The tongue consists of striated voluntary muscle and is attached mainly to the mandible and hyoid bones. The upper surface of the tongue is covered with papillae—there are three forms—the *filliform papillae* found chiefly on the dorsum of the tongue, the *fungiform* found mainly on the sides and tip of the tongue and the *vallate*—the largest of the papillae—lying in a V formation at the back of the tongue. Taste buds are resident in the walls of the vallate papillae.

There are three pairs of salivary glands, the *parotid glands* in front of and below the ears, the *sublingual glands* below the tongue and the *submandibular glands* below the mandible. The salivary glands produce secretions containing the enzyme, *ptyalin,* which helps in the digestion of cooked starches.

From the mouth the food passes into the *pharynx* which is a muscular tube that has seven openings into it. These are the *mouth*, the *oesophagus*, the *larynx*, *two posterior apertures of the nose* and *two auditory (Eustachian) tubes from the ear*.

From the pharynx the food passes into the oesophagus which is a muscular tube lined with mucous membrane and covered with fibrous tissue. From here the food passes into the stomach which is a muscular sac, its size and shape varying with its contents and muscular tone. The stomach presents two curvatures, the *greater* and the *lesser curvature* and is divided into three parts—the *cardiac portion*, the *body* and the *pyloric*. The openings into the stomach are guarded by circular bands of muscle, the *cardiac sphincter* muscle at one end and the *pyloric sphincter* muscle at the other. The stomach has three coats or coverings, the outer coat of *serous membrane*, the *middle muscular coat* and the inner *mucous membrane*. This mucous membrane is arranged in folds or rugae which disappear when the stomach is distended. The membrane is lined with glands which produce gastric juice. This contains the enzymes *pepsin* (responsible for protein digestion) and *rennin* (responsible for the curdling of milk) and also hydrochloric acid.

THE STOMACH
(anterior view)

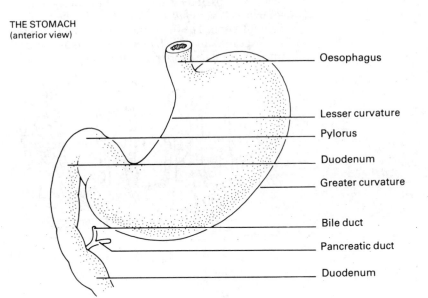

- Oesophagus
- Lesser curvature
- Pylorus
- Duodenum
- Greater curvature
- Bile duct
- Pancreatic duct
- Duodenum

From the stomach the food passes into the smaller intestine, the first part of this being the *duodenum* which is about 25 cm long and shaped like a letter 'C'. The remainder of the small intestine consists of the *jejunum* which is about 2.5 m long and the *ileum* which is about 3.5 m long. The inner coat of the small intestine is comprised of mucous membrane arranged in folds known as *valvulae conniventes* and—unlike the rugae of the stomach—these folds do not disappear with the distension of the intestines.

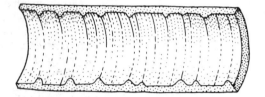

SECTION OF SMALL INTESTINE
(showing puckered lining of
valvulæ conniventes)

The mucous membrane is covered with minute fingerlike projections known as *villi*; each villus contains a lacteal for the absorption of fat and a capillary loop for the absorption of sugar and protein. This mucous membrane also contains intestinal glands which produce a secretion known as *succus entericus* which contains enzymes for the digestion of protein and sugars. The mucous membrane is studded with lymphatic nodules and, in the latter part of the small intestine, that is in the ileum, groups of these nodules are found and are known as *Peyer's patches*, their function being to fight infection. The small intestine then merges with the large intestine which though wider than the small intestine is much shorter, about 1.5 m long.

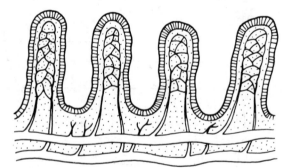

ENLARGED SECTION OF SMALL INTESTINE WALL
(showing villi)

The large intestine can be divided into nine parts; it starts with the *caecum* into which the ileum opens. The opening is guarded by the *ileo-caecal valve* which allows onflow but prevents backflow of intestinal contents. The *vermiform appendix* is attached to the blind end of the caecum and is about 7.5 cm long. The *ascending colon* passes upwards from the caecum along the right side of the abdomen and bends sharply to the left at the *right* or *hepatic flexure* to become the *transverse colon*. This passes across the abdominal cavity and turns sharply downwards at the *left* or *splenic flexure* to continue as the *descending colon*. This goes down the left side of the abdomen to the *sigmoid colon* in the pelvic cavity and the *rectum*. The rectum is about 13 cm long with 2 sphincter muscles at the exit or *anus*.

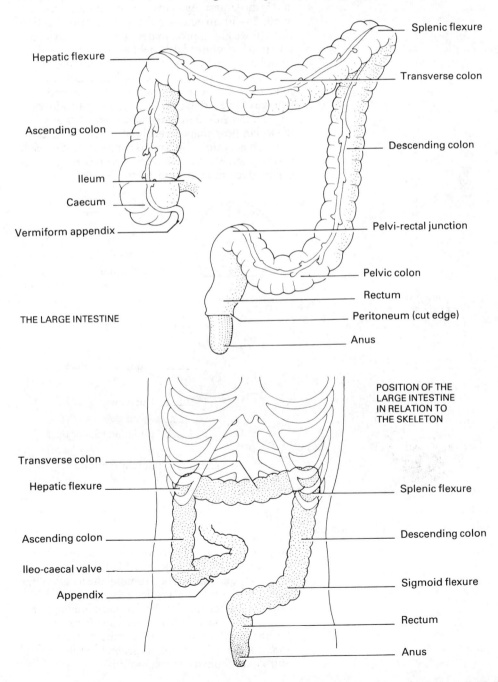

Splenic flexure

Hepatic flexure

Transverse colon

Ascending colon

Descending colon

Ileum

Caecum

Vermiform appendix

Pelvi-rectal junction

Pelvic colon

Rectum

Peritoneum (cut edge)

THE LARGE INTESTINE

Anus

POSITION OF THE
LARGE INTESTINE
IN RELATION TO
THE SKELETON

Transverse colon

Hepatic flexure

Splenic flexure

Ascending colon

Descending colon

Ileo-caecal valve

Appendix

Sigmoid flexure

Rectum

Anus

Having examined the alimentary canal it is necessary to look at the supporting organs of digestion.

The Liver

The liver is situated on the right-hand side of the body just below the diaphragm. This is really a gland and is the largest organ in the body. It measures about 25–30 cm across and 15–18 cm from back to front; it weighs approximately 1.5 kg. It is divided into two lobes—the large right lobe and the smaller left lobe. The right lobe is subdivided into the *quadrate* and *caudate* lobes. The liver has many functions and one of these is the formation and storage of bile—of which it produces up to 1 litre in a day. This passes to the gall bladder which is a muscular, pear-shaped sac about 7.5 cm long. Its function is to store bile and to concentrate it by eight to ten times; when required, the bile passes out of the gall bladder into the duodenum.

THE GALL
BLADDER AND
ITS DUCTS

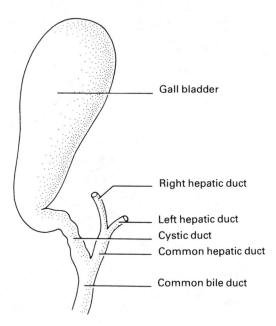

Gall bladder

Right hepatic duct

Left hepatic duct

Cystic duct

Common hepatic duct

Common bile duct

The Pancreas

The pancreas is a cream-coloured gland, 15–20 cm long and about 4 cm wide. It is divided into the head, neck, body and tail. A duct, running the length of the organ, collects pancreatic juice and passes it to the duodenum at the same point that the common bile duct passes in bile. The *islets of Langerhans* are specialised cells of the pancreas which produce *insulin*. This is passed into the general circulation and controls carbhohydrate metabolism.

ADDITIONAL NOTES ON THE PRINCIPLES OF DIGESTION

During the digestive process, large particles of protein, carbohydrate and fat are reduced in size and converted into simpler substances enabling them to be absorbed through the walls of the digestive tract into the blood stream.

Proteins are broken down to peptones and polypeptides and finally amino acids. Large particles of carbohydrates (starches or polysaccharides) are reduced to *disaccharides* which, in turn, are reduced to *monosaccharides*. Fats are split into their component parts, *fatty acids* and *glycerol*.

It should be noted that with one or two exceptions there is no absorption of food elements until they reach the intestine, where fatty acids and glycerine pass into the lacteals of the villi and amino acids into the capillary blood vessels. Fatty products are conveyed to the lymphatic system and enter the systemic circulation via the *thoracic duct*. Amino acids and simple sugars are carried by the portal vein to the liver.

The movement of food along the digestive tract is made possible by wavelike, muscular contractions known as *peristalsis*—the action is from the outside of the digestive tubes inwards and downwards, so that the food is forced further along the tube.

The stomach, being a muscularly controlled sac, is always on the move and might be compared with an old fashioned butter churn where the food is pushed around until it is well and truly mixed with gastric juice, a mixture of enzymes in hydrochloric acid.

As we have already seen, the stomach has a pyloric valve at the point where it merges into the small intestine. The function of this valve is to control the release of the partially digested food material into the small intestine. Watery foods, such as soup, leave the stomach quite quickly whilst fats remain considerably longer. An ordinary mixed diet meal is emptied from the stomach in 3–5 hours.

It has already been seen that the liver manufactures and stores bile but it has a variety of other functions. It is a powerful detoxifying organ, breaking down many kinds of toxic molecules and rendering them harmless. It is a reservoir for blood and a storage organ for some vitamins and digested carbohydrate in the form of glycogen, which it releases to sustain blood sugar levels. It manufactures enzymes, cholesterol, proteins, vitamin A from carotene, blood coagulation factors and other substances.

Bile is a complex fluid containing amongst other things bile salts and bile pigments. The pigments are derived from the disintegration of red blood cells and give the yellow brown colour of the faeces which are excreted. The bile salts are reabsorbed and reused; they promote efficient digestion of fats by a detergent action which gives very fine emulsification of fatty materials.

SOME CONDITIONS AND DISEASES OF THE DIGESTIVE SYSTEM
Appendicitis

This is an acute inflammation of the vermiform appendix. A distended, inflamed appendix may rupture—in which case it produces toxic materials and can cause peritonitis which is an acute inflammation of the abdomen.

Cirrhosis of the Liver

There are several types of cirrhosis of the liver but *portal cirrhosis* is, by far, the most common. This is also referred to as gin drinker's liver, or alcoholic liver. It is usually caused by exposure to poison, which can include such substances as carbon tetrachloride and phosphorus, but by far the most common cause is the ingestion of alcohol. This makes the liver leathery and produces nodules on its normally smooth surface—varying in size from a pin head to a bean—which give it a hobnailed appearance.

Jaundice

Jaundice is normally evidenced by the yellowness of the skin caused by an excess of bile pigments in the circulatory system. It may occur when the outflow of the bile has been blocked and when the liver surface itself is inflamed. When the small bile duct within the liver becomes obstructed a large portion of the bile which is produced by the liver is absorbed directly into the blood stream, as it cannot flow normally out of the bile duct into the duodenum.

Heartburn (Pyrosis)

This is a common sympton of gastric distress consisting of a burning sensation which extends up into the oesophagus and quite often into the throat and is accompanied by a sour belch.

Chapter 7

The Respiratory System

The respiratory system is responsible for taking in oxygen and giving off carbon dioxide and some water. It is divided into the upper respiratory tract and the lower respiratory tract. The process of taking in air into the body is *inspiration* and getting rid of air from the body is *expiration*.

THE RESPIRATORY
SYSTEM

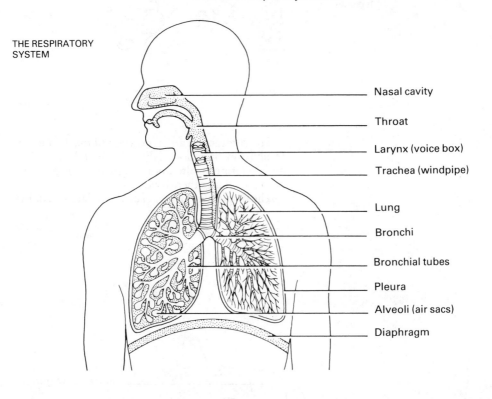

- Nasal cavity
- Throat
- Larynx (voice box)
- Trachea (windpipe)
- Lung
- Bronchi
- Bronchial tubes
- Pleura
- Alveoli (air sacs)
- Diaphragm

There are several organs involved in the respiratory system, the first being the nose. This is part of the *upper respiratory tract* which includes the mouth, the throat, the larynx and numerous sinus cavities in the head. Air brought in through the nose is filtered and warmed before passing down a tract into the lungs. The *lower respiratory tract* includes the trachea (or windpipe), the bronchi and the lungs, which contain bronchial tubes, bronchioles and alveoli, or air sacs.

The two lungs, which are the principal organs of the respiratory system, are situated in the upper part of the thoracic cage. They are inert organs, that is they do not work by themselves but function by a variation of atmospheric pressure which is achieved by a muscular wall known as the *diaphragm*.

POSITION OF THE
LUNGS WITHIN
THE THORAX

Three lobes on
right side

Two lobes on
left side

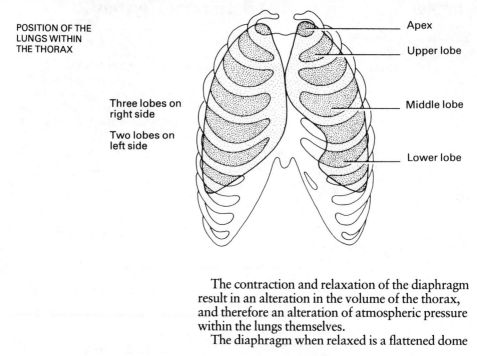

Apex

Upper lobe

Middle lobe

Lower lobe

The contraction and relaxation of the diaphragm result in an alteration in the volume of the thorax, and therefore an alteration of atmospheric pressure within the lungs themselves.

The diaphragm when relaxed is a flattened dome

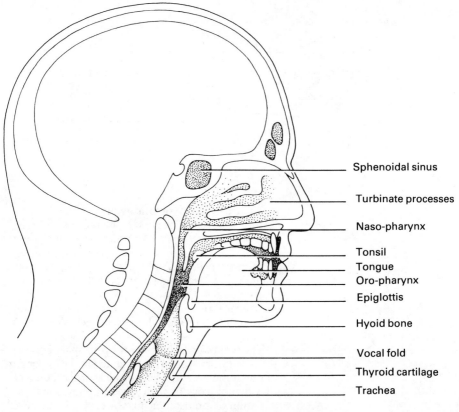

Sphenoidal sinus

Turbinate processes

Naso-pharynx

Tonsil
Tongue
Oro-pharynx
Epiglottis

Hyoid bone

Vocal fold

Thyroid cartilage

Trachea

THE UPPER RESPIRATORY PASSAGES

shape pointing upwards to the lungs. When it contracts, it flattens, pulls down the thorax, increases the volume of the thorax, and thus decreases the atmospheric pressure in the lungs. This causes air to rush in—inspiration. When the diaphragm relaxes, the thorax is pushed up, the volume decreases and the atmospheric pressure increases, and air rushes out of the lungs—expiration. The inspired air, which contains oxygen, passes down into the billions of minute air chambers or air cells known as *alveoli* which have very thin walls. Around these walls are the capillaries of the pulmonary system. It is at this point that the fresh air gives off its oxygen to the blood and takes carbon dioxide from the blood which is then expelled with the expired air.

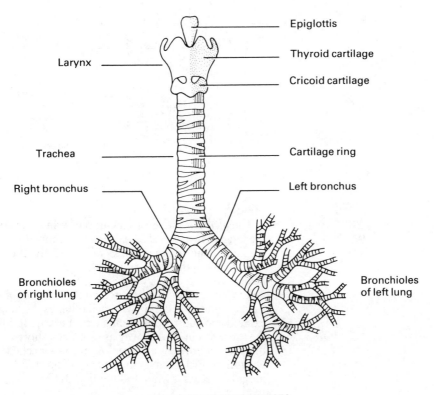

THE LOWER RESPIRATORY PASSAGES

An average adult breathes something like 13 650 litres of air a day. This is not only the body's largest intake of any substance but also the most vital. It is possible to live without food for many days, without water for a few days but without air only for a very few minutes.

The trachea or windpipe measures about 11.5 cm in length and is approximately 2.5 cm in diameter. It has rings of cartilage to prevent it collapsing. It passes through the neck in front of the oesophagus branching into two bronchi—the right bronchus being 2.5 cm long and the left bronchus 5 cm long. The bronchi branch into smaller and smaller tubes ending in the bronchioles which have no cartilage in their walls and have clusters of the thin-walled air sacs—alveoli.

The *lungs* are greyish in colour and are spongy in appearance. The right lung has three lobes—upper, middle and lower, and the left lung has two lobes—upper and lower.

SECTION OF THE
LUNG

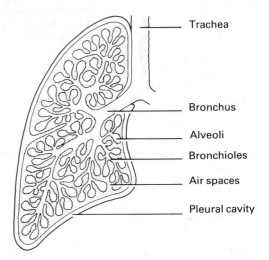

Trachea

Bronchus

Alveoli

Bronchioles

Air spaces

Pleural cavity

The *pleura* is the serous membrane which covers the lungs. The *visceral layer* is in close contact with the lung tissue and the *parietal layer* lines the chest wall. Between these layers is the *pleural cavity*. In health it is a natural cavity because the two membranes are fluid lubricated on their opposing surfaces and slide easily over each other as the lungs expand and contract. Air going into the lungs follows the same throat passageway as food for a short distance, but there is an ingenious trapdoor called the *epiglottis* which permits the passage of air to the lungs but closes it when food or liquids are swallowed.

During normal quiet breathing about 0.5 litres of air flows in and out of the lungs. This is known as *tidal air*. If inhalation is continued at the end of ordinary breathing, an additional 1.5 litres of *complemental air* can be forced into the lungs. If exhalation is continued, an extra 1.5 litres of *supplemental air* can be forced out of the lungs. About 1 litre of air remains in the lungs and cannot be expelled—this is known as *residual air*.

The normal rate of inspiration and expiration, the respiration rate, is about 16 times a minute in an adult.

CONDITIONS AND DISEASES OF THE RESPIRATORY SYSTEM

Bronchitis

This occurs in two forms—acute bronchitis and chronic bronchitis. Acute bronchitis may result from inhaled materials—fog, smoke, chemicals, etc., or it may be connected with another disease condition—influenza, measles or whooping cough. Chronic bronchitis normally occurs at middle age or later and is four times more prevalent in men than in women. The disease can prove fatal and about 30 000 deaths are recorded annually in Britain from this cause.

Pleurisy

Practically any disease that causes inflammation of the lungs may result in pleurisy. The pleura becomes inflamed and fluids accumulate in the interspace.

Pneumoconiosis

The term pneumoconiosis indicates a lung condition due to inflammation by minute particles of mineral dusts. It is often called miners' disease or miners' lung due to its prevalence amongst this body of workers. There are, however, a number of other occupations where fine dust is a hazard and workers who are exposed to a high concentration of silica dust may develop a variation of the disease known as *pneumosilicosis*. Precautionary measures like the wearing of masks help to reduce the incidence of this disease.

Pulmonary Tuberculosis

The disease we know as tuberculosis has been with us for thousands of years. Centuries before Christ it was called *Phythisis*—this is a Greek word meaning wastage or decay. This explains the familiar word for this disease—consumption. It was in 1882 that a German bacteriologist, Robert Koch, discovered that tuberculosis was caused by a long, thin bacterium called *tubercle bacillus*.

GLOSSARY

Asthma a paroxysmal condition usually due to hypersensitiveness to inhaled or ingested substances, e.g. pollen asthma.

Pneumothorax collapsed lung—may occur in accidents from bones perforating the chest. Artificial pneumothorax is the introduction of air or other gas into the pleural cavity through a needle in order to produce collapse and immobility of the lung. It is used in the treatment of pulmonary tuberculosis.

Rhinitis inflammation of the nasal mucous membrane, e.g. acute serous rhinitis—hay fever

Chapter 8

The Genito-Urinary System

In many anatomical textbooks this system is dealt with as two systems—the reproductive system and the excretive system. However, as a number of the organs involved are common to both systems the general tendency is to treat them under one heading.

The principal organs involved in the dual system are the ovaries, fallopian tubes, uterus, testes, urethra, ureter and the urinary bladder. There are a number of smaller accessory organs involved and these will be dealt with appropriately in the text.

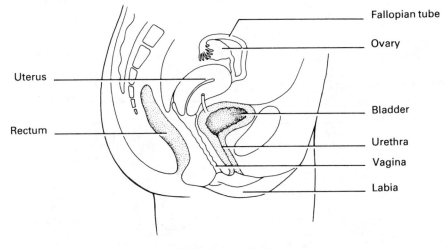

SECTION OF THE FEMALE PELVIC CAVITY

First we have the right and left *ovaries* in the female anatomy. These are quite small, about the size of an almond; they consist of masses of very small sacs known as the *ovarian follicles* and each follicle contains an egg—*ovum*. The ovaries have two principal functions:

(1) to develop the ova and expel one at approximately 28 day intervals during the reproductive life, and

(2) to produce hormones (oestrogen and progesterone) which influence secondary sex characteristics and control changes in the uterus during the menstrual cycle.

The *fallopian tubes*—sometimes referred to as the uterine tubes or oviducts—are about 10 cm long and their function is to transport the ova from the ovaries to the uterus.

The *uterus* is a muscular organ approximately

pear-shaped, about 7.5 cm long by 5 cm wide and 2.5 cm thick. It is positioned in the centre of the pelvis with the bladder in front and the rectum behind. It is normally divided into three parts—the *fundus*, the broad upper end, the *body*, the central part, and the *cervix* (about 2.5 cm long), the neck which projects into the vagina.

The *vagina* is the muscular canal which connects the above organs to the external body at the point collectively known as the *vulva* which includes the *clitoris*—a small, sensitive organ containing erectile tissue corresponding to the male penis.

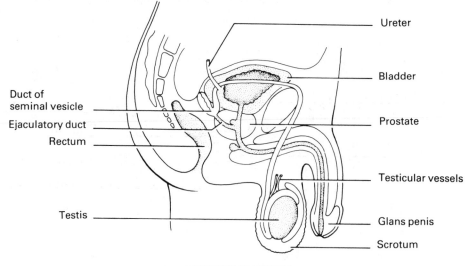

MALE GENITAL ORGANS

The male genital organs are fairly simple in comparison to the female genital organs. The principal organs are the *testes* or testicles which are the essential male reproductive glands, the *scrotum* which is a pouch-like organ containing the testes, and the *penis* which is suspended in front of the scrotum.

The *kidneys* are two bean-shaped organs, approximately 10 cm long, 5 cm wide and 2.5 cm thick. They are positioned against the posterior abdominal wall at the normal waistline, with the right kidney slightly lower than the left.

The kidneys consist of three principal parts—the *cortex* or outer layer which is light brown in colour, the *middle portion* or *medulla* which is inside and dark brown in colour and the *pelvis* which is the hollow, inner portion from which the ureters open.

The function of the kidneys is to separate certain waste products from the blood and this renal function helps maintain the blood at a constant level of composition despite the great variation in diet and fluid intake. As blood circulates in the kidneys a large

SECTION OF
KIDNEY

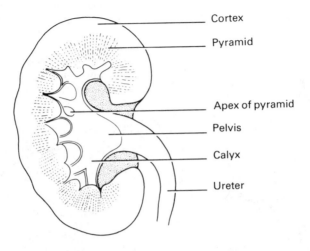

Cortex

Pyramid

Apex of pyramid

Pelvis

Calyx

Ureter

quantity of water, salts, urea and glucose is filtered into the *capsules of Bowman* and from there into the *convoluted tubules*. From here all the glucose, most of the water and salts and some of the urea are returned to the blood vessels—the remainder passes via the *calyces* into the kidney pelvis as urine. It is estimated that 150–80 litres of fluid are processed by the kidneys each day but only about 1.5 litres of this leaves the body as urine.

INTERNAL
KIDNEY
STRUCTURE

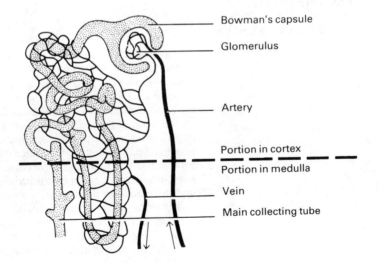

Bowman's capsule

Glomerulus

Artery

Portion in cortex

Portion in medulla

Vein

Main collecting tube

The *ureters* are two fine muscular tubes, 26–30 cm long, which carry the urine from the kidney pelvis to the bladder. This is a very elastic muscular sac lying immediately behind the *symphysis pubis*.

The *urethra* is a narrow muscular tube passing from the bladder to the exterior of the body. The female urethra is 4 cm long and the male urethra

20 cm long. In the male, the urethra is the common passage for both urine and the semen or reproductive fluid. Also, in the male, it passes through a gland known as the *prostate gland* which is about the size and shape of a chestnut. It surrounds the neck of the bladder and tends to enlarge after middle life when it may—by projecting into the bladder—produce urine retention.

THE EXCRETORY SYSTEM

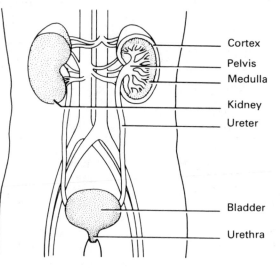

Cortex
Pelvis
Medulla
Kidney
Ureter
Bladder
Urethra

ADDITIONAL NOTES ON THE FUNCTIONS OF THE GENITO-URINARY SYSTEM

The average composition of urine is 96 per cent water and 4 per cent solid—2 per cent urea and 2 per cent salts. The 2 per cent urea compares with 0.04 per cent urea in blood plasma so it will be seen that the concentration has been increased some fifty times by the work of the kidneys. The salts consist mostly of sodium chloride, phosphates and sulphates produced partly from the presence of these salts in protein foods. These salts have either to be reabsorbed or got rid of by the kidneys in sufficient quantities to keep the normal blood balance.

The urine also contains traces of a number of other substances, all of which combine to produce in the urine a reasonable pattern of the state of the body itself. Its analysis indicates a number of physiological states including the amount of alcohol in the body, whether a female is pregnant or not and whether a person has diabetes.

It is estimated that, at birth, there are some 30 000 ova or eggs in a female child. No fresh ova are formed after birth but—during the reproductive female life—that is, commencing between 10 and 16 years of age and concluding between 45 and 55 years of age, these ova develop within the follicles or sacs in which they are embedded. They come progressively nearer to the surface of the ovary where they mature and increase in size. About every 28 days, one of these follicles bursts and the ovum it contains, together with the fluid surrounding it, is expelled into the fallopian tubes and thence into the uterus where it may or may not be fertilised. If the ovum is fertilised by a male reproductive cell or *spermatozoon* it then attaches itself to the uterine wall and develops there. If the ovum does not become fertilised within a few days it is cast off and the process termed *menstruation* is initiated.

The spermatozoa which are responsible for fertilisation are contained in a substance known as *seminal fluid*. An average ejection of seminal fluid contains several hundred million of these mobile sperm which look rather like miniature elongated tadpoles, about 0.05 mm in length. Each one consists of a headpiece, a middle piece and a long whiplike tail piece. It is this vigorous tail piece or lashing tail which gives the spermatozoon its mobility. The single fertilized ovum soon becomes many cells which develop in a bag of membranes and soon fill the uterine cavity. At one part of this sac—the point where the ovum first embedded itself in the uterine wall, the *placenta* or afterbirth develops. The umbilical cord contains blood vessels and runs from the navel of the foetus to the placenta. The placenta receives the mother's blood from the wall of the uterus and the infant's blood via the umbilical cord so that, at no stage, does the mother's blood pass directly into the child. It is through the placenta that the child's blood is able to absorb food, oxygen and water from the mother and, in turn, give off its waste products.

The skin is, of course, an organ very closely connected with the excretal system but— as it is a multipurpose organ—it is dealt with in the final chapter of this section of the book.

CONDITIONS AND DISEASES OF THE GENITO-URINARY SYSTEM

Cervicitis

This is an infection of the *cervix*, that is, the neck of the uterus, and is reasonably common. It may be due to gonorrhoea, syphilis or a specific infection.

Cystitis

Cystitis is inflammation of the bladder, a condition especially common in women. This is due to the fact that the urethra in women is very short and is a pathway to invasion by infecting organisms.

Kidney Stones

Stones in the kidney are quite common and precipitate out of the urine, which is a complex solution of many substances. Surgical operations for the removal of stones have a very long history. The Greek doctor—Hippocrates—admonished fellow physicians not to cut out stones but to leave it to the specialist. Nearer to our time, Samuel Pepys describes his own operation for the 'cutting of stone' on March 26, 1658. He notes in his diary that he spent twenty-four shillings 'for a case to keep my stone that I was cut of'.

Nephritis or Bright's Disease

This was first described by Dr Richard Bright of London in 1827. The single disease which he diagnosed has now been subdivided into a number of conditions which may, in a broader way, be called nephritis—an inflammation of the kidney not resulting from infection in the kidney.

GLOSSARY

Calculus	a stone e.g. renal calculus—stone in the kidney
Catheter	a hollow tube which is placed into a cavity through a narrow canal to discharge fluid from the cavity, e.g. draining urine from the bladder for relief of urinary retention
Dysmenorrhea	painful menstruation
Ectopic Gestation	development of the embryo in the fallopian tube instead of the uterus
Enuresis	involuntary discharge of urine
Foetus	the unborn child dating from the end of the third month until birth
Intra-uterine	within the uterus; relating to conditions which occurred before birth
Menopause	also called *climacteric*; the physiological cessation of menstruation
Micturition	the act of passing urine
Parturition	the act of giving birth

Chapter 9

The Endocrine System

Hormones are chemicals which cause certain changes in particular parts of the body. Their effects are slower and more general than nerve action. They can control long-term changes such as rate of growth, rate of activity and sexual maturity.

The *endocrine* or *ductless glands* secrete their hormones directly into the blood stream. The hormones are circulated all over the body and reach their target organ via the blood stream. When hormones pass through the liver, they are converted into relatively inactive compounds which are excreted by the kidneys. Tests on such hormonal end products in urine can be used to detect pregnancy.

The *endocrine system* consists of a series of glands which secrete hormones; they are found throughout the body and include the pituitary, thyroid, parathyroids, thymus, supra-renal or adrenal glands, part of the pancreas and parts of the ovaries and testes.

Although these glands are separate—it is certain that they are functionally closely related because the health of the body is dependent upon the correctly balanced output from the various glands that form this system.

The Pituitary Gland (Hypophysis)

This gland has been described as the leader of the endocrine orchestra. It consists of two lobes, anterior and posterior. The anterior lobe secretes many hormones, including the growth-promoting *somatotropic* hormone which controls the bones and muscles and in this way determines the overall size of the individual. Oversecretion of the hormone in children produces gigantism and undersecretion produces dwarfism. The anterior lobe also produces *gonadotropic* hormones for both male and female gonad activity. *Thyrotropic* hormones regulate the thyroid and *adrenocorticotropic* hormones regulate the adrenal cortex. It also produces *metabolic* hormones.

The posterior lobe produces two hormones— *oxytocin* and *vasopressin*. Oxytocin causes the uterine muscles to contract; it also causes the ducts of the mammary glands to contract and, in this way, helps to express the milk which the gland has secreted into the ducts. Vasopressin is an antidiuretic hormone which has a direct effect on the tubules of the kidneys and increases the amount of fluid they absorb so that less urine is excreted. It also contracts blood vessels in the heart and lungs and so raises the blood pressure. It is not certain whether these two hormones are actually manufactured in the posterior lobe or whether they are produced in the hypothalamus and passed down the stalk of the pituitary gland to be stored in the posterior lobe and liberated from there into the circulation.

The Thyroid

The right and left lobes of this gland lie on either side of the *trachea* united by the *isthmus*. The average size of each lobe is 4 cm long and 2 cm across but these sizes may vary considerably. The secretion of this gland is *thyroxine* and *tri-iodothyronine*. Thyroxine controls the general metabolism. Both hormones contain iodine but thyrónine is more active than thyroxin. Under-secretion of this hormone in children produces cretinism; the children show

GLANDS OF THE BODY

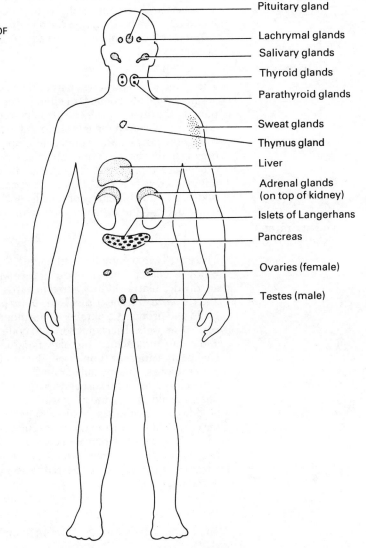

- Pituitary gland
- Lachrymal glands
- Salivary glands
- Thyroid glands
- Parathyroid glands
- Sweat glands
- Thymus gland
- Liver
- Adrenal glands (on top of kidney)
- Islets of Langerhans
- Pancreas
- Ovaries (female)
- Testes (male)

stunted growth (dwarfism) and fail to develop mentally. Undersecretion in adults results in a low metabolic rate. Oversecretion in adults gives rise to exophthalmic goitre and the metabolic rate is higher than usual. Such persons may eat well but burn up so much fuel that they remain thin. This is usually accompanied by a rapid pulse rate. This gland, therefore, has a profound influence on both mental and physical activity.

The Parathyroid Glands

There are four of these glands, two on either side lying behind the thyroid. Their secretion is *parathormone*—the function of which is to raise the blood calcium as well as maintain the balance of calcium and phosphorus in both the blood and bone structures. Undersecretion gives rise to a condition known as *tetany* in which the muscles go into spasm, and oversecretion causes calcium to be lost to the blood from the bones giving rise to softened bones, raised blood calcium and a marked depression of the nervous system.

The Thymus Gland

This gland lies in the lower part of the neck and attains a maximum length of about 6 cm. After puberty the thymus begins to atrophy so that in the adult only fibrous remnants are found. Its secretion is thought to act as a brake on the development of sex organs so that as the thymus atrophies, the sex organs develop. Recent research into the activity of this gland reveals that it plays an important part in the body's immune system by producing T lymphocytes—the T standing for thymus derived.

The Suprarenal or Adrenal Glands

These are two in number, triangular in shape and yellow in colour. They lie one over each kidney. They are divided like the kidney into two parts—the *cortex* and the *medulla*. The cortex is the outer part of the gland and produces a number of hormones called *cortico-steroids*. Their function is to control sodium and potassium balance, stimulate the storage of glucose and affect or supplement the production of sex hormones. The medulla or inner layer produces *adrenalin*, a powerful vasoconstrictor. Adrenalin raises the blood pressure by constriction of smaller blood vessels and raises the blood sugar by increasing the output of sugar from the liver. The amount of adrenalin secreted is increased considerably by excitement, fear, or anger, which has caused the adrenals sometimes to be referred to as the glands of fright and fight.

The Gonads or Sex Glands

These glands are naturally different in men and

women because they serve different, though, in many respects, complementary functions. In the female the gonads are the ovaries and in the male the testes. Female sex hormones are *oestrogen* and *progesterone*. The male sex hormone is *testosterone*, though each sex produces a small quantity of the opposite hormone. The female hormones are responsible for developing the rounded, feminine figure, breast growth, pubic and axillary hair and all the normal manifestations of femininity and reproduction. Male hormone is responsible for voice changes, increased muscle mass, development of hair on the body and face and the usual development of manliness.

Pancreas

The endocrine part of the pancreas consists of clumps of cells called *islets of Langerhans* which secrete *insulin*. Insulin regulates the sugar level in the blood and the conversion of sugar into heat and energy. Too little insulin results in a disease known as *diabetes mellitus*. This disease is divided into one form, juvenile onset, which occurs before the age of 25, and another form which begins in maturity. It is a very common disease. It is known that some half million people in the United Kingdom suffer from it sufficiently badly to need treatment but it has been estimated that there are many more people in whom the disease exists at a sub-treatment level. Drs Rankin and Best succeeded in 1922 in keeping a diabetic dog alive in their Canadian laboratory by injection of insulin. More recently, with surgery, it has been possible to contain this disease although the supplement of insulin is really a support treatment rather than a cure.

ADDITIONAL NOTES ON THE HORMONE SYSTEM

The quantities involved in the secretion of the various glands are minute. For example, the adrenal glands, which affect all the organs of the body, produce in a complete year not more than 1 g of hormone. Some hormone deficiencies appear to be endemic, that is they are particularly prevalent in certain parts of the world. The best example is probably to be found in the diseases which affect the thyroid through lack of iodine. For example, endemic cretinism is common to the upper valleys of the Alps and the Himalayas where endemic goitre is also present, whilst the latter condition is to be found also in the region of the Great Lakes and the Valley of Saint Lawrence. In all these areas, which are deficient in iodine or iodine-containing foods, the authorities now usually take precautionary measures such as the provision of iodised salts in order to stop the development of the disease.

GLOSSARY

Addison's Syndrome   a condition due to adrenal cortical tissue insufficiency, characterised by hypotension, wasting, vomiting and muscular weakness

Amenorrhoea   absence of menstruation

Cushing's Syndrome   condition due to oversecretion of adreno-cortical hormones, characterised by moon face, redistribution of body fat, hypertension, muscular weakness and occasionally mental derangement

Hyperthyroidism   thyrotoxicosis, toxic goitre and Graves' disease or exophthalmic goitre: the body's physical activities are subject to a speeding up whilst the opposite condition—hypothyroidism—is evidenced by a slowing down of the body's activities

Lesion   an alteration of structure or of functional capacity due to injury or disease.

Menopause (Climacteric)   cessation of menses; the period in female development when the reproductive function comes to an end, linked to a decline in the supply of hormone secretions by the ovaries. This is not a disease—it marks another stage in the female progression through life

Premenstrual Tension   a syndrome of depression, irritability, bloating, swelling and restlessness that occurs for about one week before the onset of menstruation

Steroid   the generic name given to various compounds of internal secretions including the sex hormones

Syndrome   a group of symptoms and signs which, when considered together, characterise a disease

Chapter 10

Accessory Organs

The subject title of this chapter describes those parts of the human anatomy which do not fit completely into any one system although they may form part of it.

THE SKIN

The skin is an important organ which has three primary functions:

(1) It serves as a protective cover.
(2) It regulates body temperature.
(3) It provides a sensory covering over the entire body.

It has two principal divisions, the epidermis or outer skin and the dermis or true skin.

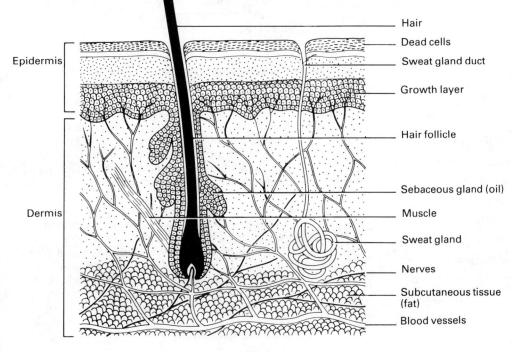

THE SKIN

Skin is a large organ. The average human adult is covered by about 1.7 m² of skin, varying in thickness from thin over the eyelids to thick on the soles of the feet. It weighs about 3.2 kg and provides an excellent protection against germs as very few can penetrate unbroken skin. Normal body processes produce heat and most of this is eliminated from the skin by radiation to the surrounding air or by evaporation of perspiration.

As an indication of the complexity of the skin it has been estimated that 1 cm^2 of skin contains approximately 3 million cells, 13 oil glands, 9 hairs, 100 sweat glands, 2.75 m of nerves, 1 m of blood vessels and thousands of sensory cells. It is, therefore, easy to see how healthy skin is indicative of good mental and physical health.

The *epidermis* is the outer layer of the skin which contains nerve endings but no blood vessels. It is nourished by tissue fluid derived from the dermis.

The *dermis* is a thicker layer of connective tissue which supports the hairs, each hair growing from a hair follicle.

The *erector pili* muscles, which are attached to the hair follicles, contract in response to cold and fear.

The *sebaceous glands* secrete sebum; *sweat* or *sudoriferous glands* extract water, salts, urea and other waste products and discharge them on to the skin surface as sweat.

Sensory nerve endings give sensations of touch, pain and temperature; superficial blood vessels play a part in regulating body temperature.

Nails are really appendages of the skin, being outgrowths from the epidermis.

Adipose tissue beneath the skin is one of the principal fat deposits of the body.

The *sweat glands* of the skin are of two types. The first produce *apocrine sweat* which has more social than physiological significance. The apocrine sweat glands are limited to a few regions of the body, primarily the axillary and genital areas. They are inactive in infants, develop with puberty and enlarge premenstrually. Freshly produced sweat is normally sterile and inoffensive but its decomposition by bacteria gives rise to perspiration odour.

The second kind of sweat is called *eccrine*—there are millions of these sweat glands all over the body and the sweat they give out is little more than diluted salt water. They are involved in the vital heat regulating system that enables the body to keep its constant internal temperature at 36.8°C. These eccrine sweat glands disperse large quantities of water which, in extreme circumstances, can reach as much as 2.3 litres a day.

THE EYES

Our sense of sight is the response of the brain to light stimuli which are received through the eye. The eyeball is a hollow, spherical structure, its walls consisting of three principal layers:

(1) The *sclera* is a tough fibrous, opaque coat, which is modified in front to form the clear, transparent *cornea*.
(2) The *choroid* or middle coat consists of an interlacement of blood vessels and pigment

granules supported by loose connective tissue;
the *iris* is a pigmented, muscular curtain
suspended behind the cornea. In the centre of the
iris is an aperture known as the *pupil* through
which light reaches the interior of the eye.

(3) The *retina* forms the delicate inner layer of the
eyeball. In this layer are found the *receptor* and
sensory optic nerve endings sometimes referred
to as *rods* and *cones*.

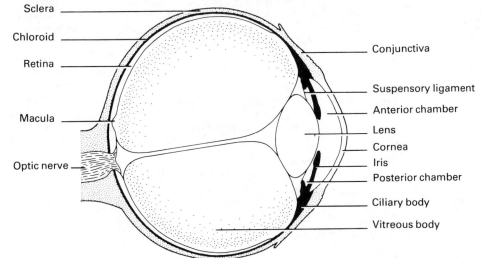

THE EYEBALL

The eyeball has a number of appendages; the
various muscles which directionally rotate it and
the *lachrymal* or *tear glands* which moisten and
clean the outer surface of the eye. Excess
secretion of the lachrymal glands overflows onto
the cheeks as tears. From the inner corners of the
eyes the tears drain into a channel which opens
into the nose, which is why weeping is sometimes
accompanied by sniffing.

The pupil controls the light image by
contracting in bright light and dilating in dim
light. These light images strike the retina as an
upside down image which is then conveyed to
the brain through the optic nerve. The brain then
reinverts the impulse so that it becomes a right
side up image.

THE EARS

The ear is made up of three parts—the *external* ear,
the *middle* ear and the *internal* ear.

(1) **The external ear** consists of the *auricle* attached
to the side of the head and the *external auditory
meatus* leading from the auricle (or *pinna*) to the
tympanic membrane or ear-drum. The function
of the auricle is to collect sound waves and
conduct them to the external auditory canal and

tympanic membrane. The external auditory meatus or canal contains ceruminous glands which secrete cerumen or wax.

(2) *The middle ear* or *tympanic cavity* is a small air-filled cavity containing a chain of small bones—*auditory ossicles*. Sound waves are transmitted from the tympanic membrane (parchment-like) by the auditory bones (malleus, incus and stapes, popularly known as the hammer, anvil and stirrup) to the oval window (*fenestra ovalis*), a membrane connecting with the internal ear.

The *Eustachian* (*auditory*) *tube* links the ear with the nasopharynx to ensure that air pressure in the middle ear is the same as atmospheric pressure. The middle ear also communicates with the *mastoid antrum* and mastoid air cells in the mastoid process of the temporal bone.

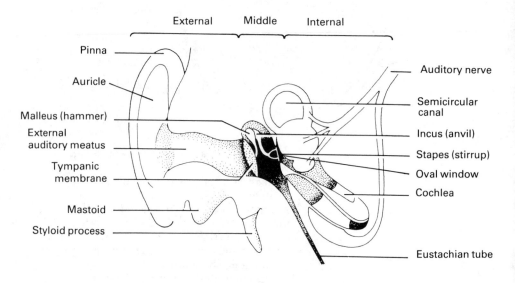

A SECTION THROUGH THE EAR

(3) *The internal ear* or *labyrinth* consists of bony cavities (*osseous labyrinth*) enclosing a membranous structure (*membranous labyrinth*) which approximately follows the shape of the bony labyrinth. Between the bony walls and the membranous part of the labyrinth is a clear fluid—*perilymph*. This transmits the vibrations from the oval window to the *cochlea* (the essential organ of hearing) which connects to the brain via the auditory nerve. The *three semi-circular* canals (membranous canals or ducts) are situated in the bony labyrinth and control balance.

THE MAMMARY GLANDS OR BREASTS

These are accessories to the female reproductive organs and secrete milk during the period of lactation. They enlarge at puberty, increase in size during pregnancy and atrophy in old age. The breast consists of mammary gland substance or *alveolar* tissue arranged in lobes and separated by connective and fatty tissues. Each lobule consists of a cluster of alveoli opening into lactiferous ducts which unite with other ducts to form large ducts which terminate in the excretory ducts. The ducts near the nipple expand to create reservoirs for the milk—*lactiferous sinuses*.

The breast contains a considerable quantity of fat, which lies in the tissue of the breast and also in between the lobes. It contains numerous lymphatic vessels which commence as tiny plexuses, unite to form larger vessels and eventually pass mainly to the lymph node in the axilla. The nipple is surrounded by a darker coloured area known as the mammary areola.

The breasts are greatly influenced by hormone activity. Hyper-secretion of the thyroid can lead to atrophy of the breasts while hypo-secretion can cause greatly developed breasts. Both the ovarian hormones influence the condition and appearance of the breast whilst the pituitary hormone, *prolactin*, starts lactation at the end of pregnancy.

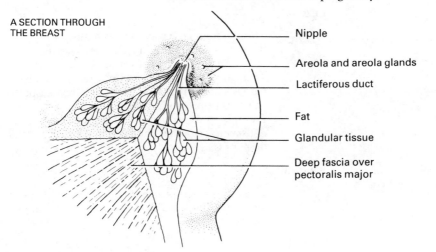

A SECTION THROUGH THE BREAST

Nipple

Areola and areola glands

Lactiferous duct

Fat

Glandular tissue

Deep fascia over pectoralis major

CONDITIONS AND DISEASES OF THE ACCESSORY ORGANS

Acne Vulgaris or Common Acne

This is one of the most common forms of skin disease. It is due to an oversecretion of the sebaceous glands and is invariably associated with the increase of sex hormones at puberty in both male and female. The primary lesion of acne is the *comedo* or *blackhead*, the blackhead being darkened by air and not by dirt as sometimes thought.

Alopecia Areata (patchy baldness)

In this condition hair is lost from a small area, generally on the scalp but sometimes in the hirsute area of the face. There is no inflammation or any obvious skin disorder or systemic disease.

Cataract

The lens of the eye is situated directly behind the pupil and in health is clear. With age and in some diseases such as diabetes it loses its transparency and becomes more opaque, gradually shutting out vision—this condition is known as a cataract. It is not a growth but a biochemical change in the lens.

Conjunctivitis

This is inflammation of the conjunctiva. In its acute contagious form it is known as 'Pink Eye'. It is caused by various forms of bacterial and viral infections. It includes swimming pool conjunctivitis and the type which is developed as a result of exposure to ultraviolet rays.

Eczema

This is a term now used synonymously with dermatitis. It is not so much a disease as a complex symptom with many causes and clinical variations. There are a number of types or categories, their names—in many cases—indicating their suspected environmental or physiological cause. For example—lipstick dermatitis, perfume dermatitis, housewife's eczema (hand eczema) and industrial dermatitis.

Keloids

These are rather like elevated scars and can occur after burns, cuts, scalds or surgical wounds anywhere on the skin.

Psoriasis

Psoriasis is a common form of skin disease estimated to affect some five or six per cent of the population. It affects both sexes and is more commonly found in adults than children. It occurs in families sometimes and in about 25 per cent of cases it is hereditary. Psoriasis is characterised by the development of elevated reddish patches covered by a thick, dry, silvery scale.

Stye or Hordeolum

A stye or hordeolum is usually caused by bacteria getting into the roots of one or more of the eyelashes, where local infection takes place. If, on the other hand, the infection gets into the sweat glands of the eyelid—a *cyst* or *chalazion* forms.

Tineacapitis (Ringworm of the Scalp)

This superficial fungus infection of the scalp occurs in male or female before puberty and is characterised by partial loss of scalp hair and the breaking off of infected hairs. It is spread by direct contact with an infected person or through the use of a comb or headgear that has been worn by an infected person.

Verruca (Warts)

There are many types of verruca, the best known being *verruca vulgaris* or common wart and *verruca plantaris* which occurs on the soles of the feet. They are a dry, elevated lesion which may appear singly or in large numbers. They are caused by viruses.

GLOSSARY

Acne Rosacea	unrelated to common acne; a chronic disease which affects the skin of the middle third of the face. It occurs most frequently in middle-aged women in whom it is associated with intestinal disturbances or pelvic disease
Antrum	a cavity or hollow space in a bone
Auditory Vertigo	dizziness due to disease of the ears
Blister	a collection of fluid between the epidermis and the dermis
Colour Blindness	a congenital inherited condition passed down by the female carriers to their sons
Hirsutism	a condition characterised by growth of hair in unusual places and in unusual amounts
Ocular Vertigo	dizziness due to disease of the eyes
Tinea Pedis (Athlete's Foot)	a fungal infection which is more common in men and more frequent in summer. In the acute form the blister type is the most common
Vertigo	giddiness; sensation of loss of equilibrium
Vesicle	a small sac containing fluid—a skin blister

Chapter 11

Histology

Histology can be readily defined in two words—microscopic anatomy. It is the branch of biology which deals with the minute structure of tissues which are the basis of cell life.

All living structures are composed of cells and intercellular material. Some of this intercellular material provides strength, for example, collagen and elastic fibres in the skin and calcium salts in the bone, whilst much of the intercellular material acts as a cement between the cells. This is sometimes referred to as *ground substance* or *interstitial substance*.

Life starts when a single ovum (female sex cell) is fertilised by a spermatozoon (male sex cell). These sex cells are formed by a process, meiosis, in which the number of *chromosomes* (genetic material) in the nucleus is halved.

This fertilised cell consists of a nucleus, containing the full complement of chromosomes, surrounded by protoplasm and enclosed by a membrane. It divides by a process called mitosis, in which the essential elements of the nucleus, the chromosomes, are reproduced in each daughter cell. The chromosomes are made up of a linear arrangement of genes. It is now known that the genes in each cell (*genome*) contain a complete pattern of the human body.

In 1943 it was discovered that genes were made from very long, large molecules of *deoxyribonucleic acid*, DNA for short, but the way in which DNA carried all the information to produce a complete human being remained unknown until 1953. It was then discovered that DNA was made of four different small molecules called *nucleotides* linked together in a long chain. The most important feature of DNA is that two of these very long chains twist around each other to form a double helix rather like a rubber ladder twisted around its long axis. The DNA molecule is by far the largest molecule found in the cell, which is not surprising, considering the amount of information it has to carry in its four letter alphabet.

In each cell there are something like 30 000 million such letters, equivalent to 1000 books of 1000 pages each. It will be seen that the genes carry the determining factors of inheritance and cell behaviour.

Gradually, as a result of mitosis, a ball of cells is formed and in the very early stages this ball of cells can be divided into three layers:

(1) An outer layer—the *ectoderm* or *epiblast* from which the skin, its appendages and the nervous system are developed.
(2) A middle layer—the *mesoderm* or *mesoblast*

from which fat and various internal organs are developed.

(3) An inner layer—the *endoblast* which provides the lining of a number of organs of the body.

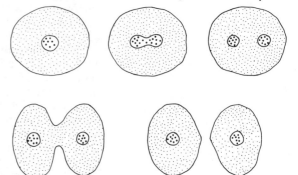

CELL MITOSIS

So the single cell has developed into tissue and, when fully developed, there are four types of tissue in the body:

(1) **The Epithelium**
(2) **Connective Tissue**
(3) **Muscular Tissue**
(4) **Nerve Tissue**

Epithelium

The epithelium is divided into two principal varieties:

a. *Simple epithelium* which consists of one layer of cells. It is very delicate and is found in several organ linings like the thorax and the abdomen.

b. *Stratified* or *compound epithelium* which consists of two or more layers.

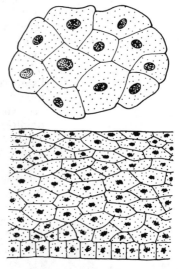

Connective Tissue

This connects all other tissues and when presented in the form of bone gives support and rigidity to the body. There are seven principal varieties of

CONNECTIVE
TISSUE

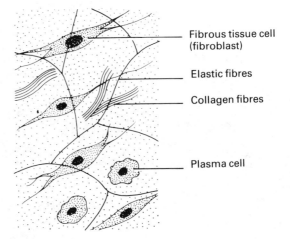

Fibrous tissue cell
(fibroblast)

Elastic fibres

Collagen fibres

Plasma cell

connective tissue:
(1) Areolar or loose connective tissue—this forms a
    very thin transparent tissue which surrounds
    vessels, nerves and muscle fibres.
(2) Adipose tissue—this is not unlike loose
    connective tissue but the spaces of the network
    are filled in with fat cells.

FAT CELLS BOUNDED
BY WHITE CONNECTIVE
TISSUE FIBRES

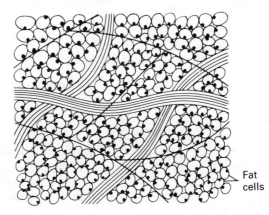

Fat
cells

(3) Fibrous tissue—this is found in tendons and
    ligaments and also forms the outside of various
    organs such as the kidney and heart, as well as
    the outside of bone and muscle.
(4) Bone—this is a special type of fibrous material
    hardened by the deposit of such salts as calcium
    phosphate, the fibrous material giving it
    toughness and the mineral matter giving it
    rigidity.
(5) Cartilage—this is a specialised type of fibrous
    tissue. It is tough and pliable and very strong. It
    provides a firm wall to the larynx and the trachea

and for the pads which join bone to bone in the slightly movable joints, for example between the vertebrae.

(6) Yellow elastic tissue—found where elasticity is important as in the walls of blood vessels.

(7) Lymphoid or reticular—found in lymph nodes and the spleen.

WHITE
FIBROCARTILAGE

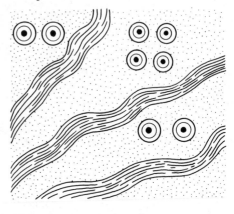

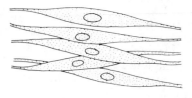

SMOOTH MUSCLE FIBRE

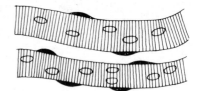

STRIATED MUSCLE FIBRE

Muscular tissue

This is contractile tissue and is able to produce movement. This is dealt with in more detail in the chapter 'The Muscular System'.

Nerve tissue

This has the special function of carrying messages or stimuli throughout the body. It consists of nerve cells and nerve fibres and is dealt with in greater detail under the heading 'The Neurological System'.

NERVE TISSUE

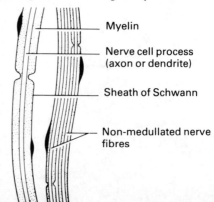

— Myelin

— Nerve cell process (axon or dendrite)

— Sheath of Schwann

— Non-medullated nerve fibres

In addition to these there are three liquid or fluid tissues—the *blood*, *lymph* and *cerebro-spinal fluid*. Each of these is dealt with under the appropriate heading.

Membranes

These are made of connective tissue and line the cavities and hollow organs of the body. They secrete lubricating fluids to moisten their smooth surfaces and prevent friction. There are three types of membrane found in the human body:

(1) Synovial membrane secretes a very thick fluid rather like egg white in consistency.
(2) Mucous membrane secrets a sticky fluid called *mucus*.
(3) Serous membrane is made of flattened cells through which a small quantity of a thin, watery substance oozes. The fluid which emanates from it is called *serum*.

Waterlogging of the tissues can occur and when this happens it is called *oedema*. This can arise from a number of causes:

(1) Too high hydrostatic pressure in the capillaries.
(2) An osmotic pressure that is too low.
(3) A blockage of lymphatic vessels.
(4) Damage to the capillary walls.

Cardiac oedema is the type which occurs in congestive heart trouble and this is caused by the increase in venous pressure and the consequent increase in capillary pressure. It is characterised by swelling of the legs and feet of those who habitually walk or stand whilst it appears in the lower part of the back or buttocks of those who lie. An important factor is the kidneys and their diminished secretion of sodium.

SUMMARY

Human beings start as a single cell formed by the fusion of two sex cells.

Mitosis is the principle or method used by the cell for multiplication. Most tissues are dealt with under their respective headings but this chapter has primarily been concerned with connective tissue which serves as the supporting system of the body. Its cells are responsible for the elements and matrix of bone, cartilaginous and fibrous tissue. They form the various tough frameworks of the body whilst the matrix supplies lubricating elements which facilitate easy movement.

Collagen was, at one time, used synonymously with connective tissue but is now used more specifically to indicate connective tissue fibres.

Ground substance is a type of cementing material found between the minute fibres and binding them together.

GLOSSARY

Centrosome	a very small, dense part of the cytoplasm lying close to the nucleus
Chromosomes	thread-shaped bodies consisting of DNA, found in the nucleus of the cell. There are 23 pairs (46 in total) in each human cell
Genes	hereditary determinants occurring in the chromosomes in linear arrangement
Grand Cytoplasm	a type of protoplasm surrounding the nucleus, in which the other structures are embedded
Golgi Apparatus	a canal-like structure lying close to the nucleus; named after the famous Italian histologist who first described it at the beginning of this century
Karyokinesis	same as mitosis—cell division
Meiosis	the type of cell division which takes place in the sex organs. The number of chromosomes is halved so that a spermatazoon provides 23 chromosomes and the ovum 23 chromosomes
Mitochondria	small, rodlike structures embedded in the cytoplasm
Pathology	a branch of science which deals with the nature of disease through the study of cause, process, effect and associated alterations of structure and function

GENERAL GLOSSARY OF ANATOMY AND PHYSIOLOGY

Acute   having rapid onset, a short course with pronounced symptoms

Anastomosis   the intercommunication of the vessels of any system with one another

Ankylosis   stiffness or fixation of a joint

Aplasia   absence of growth

Aponeurosis   the white, shiny membrane covering the muscles or connecting the muscles and tendons with the parts they move

Asthenia   the absence of strength in the muscles

Astigmatism   a defect in the focusing apparatus of the eyes

Benign   a tumour which is not malignant

Bilateral   on both sides

Biopsy   microscopic examination of tissue taken from a living subject

Calorie   a unit of heat that is the amount which raises the temperature of 1 kilogramme of water 1 °C

Cardiologist   medically qualified person who specialises in the diagnosis and treatment of disorders of the heart and vascular system

Catalyst   a substance which greatly increases the rate of chemical reaction

Chronic   of long duration—opposite to acute

Condyle   rounded projection at the end of a bone, forming part of a joint with another bone

Costal   relating to the ribs

Digit   finger or toe

Displasia   disordered growth

Dorsum   any part corresponding to the back, e.g. dorsum of the tongue

Dyspnoea   difficulty of breathing

Enzyme   a catalytic substance having a specific action in promoting a chemical change

Effusion   an abnormal outpouring of fluid (serum, pus or blood) into the tissues or cavities of the body

Electrocardiogram (ECG)   a graphic recording of the electric potential differences due to cardiac action taken from the body surfaces

Electroencephalogram (EEG)   a graphic recording of the minute changes in the electric potential associated with brain activity as detected by electrodes applied to the scalp surface

Filiform	slender—like a thread
Follicle	a small tubular or sac-like depression
Foramen	a hole
Fungiform	having a shape similar to that of a mushroom
Fusiform	spindle-shaped, tapering both ways like a spindle
Gallstones	constituents of gall bladder which have crystallised
Glomerulus	a cluster of capillary vessels in the kidney
Hemiplegia	paralysis of half the body divided vertically
Hepatic	pertaining to the liver
Ingestion	the taking in of food
Keratin	proteins, the chief constituent of nails and hair
Lobe	a rounded part or projection of an organ
Lobule	a small lobe
Matrix	that which encloses anything
Melanin	pigment found in the cells of the skin
Micturition	the act of passing urine
Mitral Valve	the heart valve between the atrium or auricle and ventricle
Myopia	short or near sight
Neoplasm	new growth
Neuroglia	connective tissue of the central nervous system
Neurologist	medically qualified person specialising in the diagnosis and treatment of disorders of the nervous system
Olfactory	pertaining to the sense of smell
Optic	relating to the sense of vision
Orthopaedic Surgeon	a person who is medically qualified and specialises in that branch of surgery devoted to the prevention and correction of bone deformities
Osmosis	the diffusion of liquid substances through membranes
Osseous	bony or composed of bones
Paraplegia	paralysis of half the body divided horizontally
Pathogenic	disease producing
Periphery	circumference; an external surface; the parts away from the centre
Peritoneum	the serous membrane lining the interior of the abdominal cavity
Physiatrist	a person who is specially trained in physical therapy especially for the promotion of health and fitness

Physiotherapist	a person who is specially trained in the science and art of physical medicine
Plexus	an intricate network of nerves, veins or lymphatic vessels
Psychiatrist	a person who is medically qualified and has specialised in mental or psychological conditions
Psychology	the science of the study of the structure and function of the mind; the behaviour of an organism in relation to its environment
Psychosomatic	a body/mind relationship
Pus	the thick white, yellow or greenish fluid found in abscesses, on ulcers or on inflamed and discharging surfaces, composed largely of dead white blood cells
Renal	pertaining to the kidneys
Retina	the innermost and light-sensitive coat of the eyeball
Sarcoma	a malignant tumour composed of cells derived from non-epithelial tissue, mainly connective tissues
Somatic	relating to the body
Squamous	scaly or shaped like a scale
Stenosis	contraction or narrowing of a channel or opening
Symphysis	the line of junction of two bones
Tactile	pertaining to touch or touch sensation
Tricuspid Valve	valve of the heart guarding the passage from the right atrium or auricle to the ventricle
Tuberosity	a protuberance on a bone
Unilateral	on one side
Vasconstrictor	a nerve causing constriction of a blood vessel
Vasodilator	a nerve causing dilation of a blood vessel

PART II

The Study and Application of Therapy Treatments

In no way does this section pretend to be an exhaustive study of the subjects under review, but rather an attempt to spell out the main principles involved in such a way that the student is able to relate the value of one treatment to another in a particular circumstance, or know how best to combine treatments in a way which will be the most satisfactory.

Most of the subjects under review have had many books written about them and in much greater detail than is possible in a textbook of this kind.

Students who wish to research more deeply into any one particular subject have at their disposal a large bibliography from which to choose, but the following chapters will give the student a good grounding in the use of some of the more popular treatments in physical therapy.

Chapter 12

Massage

It is generally believed that the word *massage* derives from the Arabic 'mass' or 'Mas'h' meaning to press softly. As an art it must be about as old as man himself because to hold or rub an injured part is an instinctive reaction to the pain involved. We know from ancient writings that the Chinese had a system of massage at least 5000 years ago—as did the Hindus, the Japanese and, just a little nearer our time, the ancient Egyptians.

In the far off days massage, as an integral adjunct to medicine, was largely practised by the priest/doctor, and many people believe that the laying on of hands, rather than being a religious ceremony, was a practical application by the priest for the relief of pain and the acceleration of health in the tissues.

There are a number of incidents in the Bible and other holy books which may be interpreted in this way. Amongst the very early writings it is interesting to note that 3000 years before the Christian era, Chinese priests said in the Kong-Fu—'Early morning effleurage with the palm of the hand, after a night's sleep when the blood is rested and the temper more relaxed, protects against cold, keeps the organs supple and prevents many minor ailments'. Or again, about the same time, the Hindu priests were writing—'massage reduces fat, strengthens the muscles and firms the skin'.

However, it is to the writers of the Greek dynasty that we are most indebted for early records of the way in which massage was used as an important part of the system of medicine. In the year 380 BC, Hippocrates wrote 'A physician must be experienced in many things but assuredly also in rubbing—for things that have the same names have not always the same effect, for rubbing can bind a joint that is too loose and loosen a joint that is too tight; rubbing can bind and loosen; can make flesh or cause parts to waste; hard rubbing binds, soft rubbing loosens. Much rubbing causes parts to waste, moderate rubbing makes them grow'.

This medicinal use of massage appears to have been transferred to the Roman Empire because the famous physician—Galen, who lived during the 2nd century AD in Rome, was an advocate of massage in the treatment of injuries and certain diseases. He wrote 'Massage eliminates the waste products of nutrition and the poisons of fatigue'. However, with the decline of the Roman Empire, it would appear that massage became less associated with medicine and more with the pursuit of pleasure so that massage, rather than being something that was practised by the physicians and their trained assistants, was an art applied to the Romans by their slaves as a substitute for strenuous exercise and to help reduce the effects of excessive eating and drinking.

During the dark days of the Middle Ages the scientific use of massage largely disappeared though a general understanding of human nature suggests that it must have been practised in some form or other during these times and it may be that the only weak link in the chain is the lack of documentary reference for most of that era. It reappears again in writings in the 16th century.

In the early 19th century a Swede, by the name of Ling, developed a scientific system of massage and exercise based on physiology. It is to Henreich Ling, who died in 1839, that we are indebted for our modern concept of Swedish massage though many years were to pass before it was generally accepted by the medical profession as a form of treatment and it was not until 1899 that Sir William Bennett inaugurated a Massage Department at St. George's Hospital, London.

SWEDISH MASSAGE

Swedish massage may be defined as the manipulation of soft tissue for therapeutic purposes. It is traditionally performed with talc powder and this is applied to the hands of the therapist (not shaken on to the patient), as its aim is to enable the therapist's hands to slide over the patient. Putting talc on the patient results in the movements of massage forcing small particles into the pores thereby inhibiting some of the effects which should be achieved.

Massage has both a physiological and a psychological effect. The various movements massage exerts, either individually or in combination, affect the skin, muscle, blood vessels, lymphatics, nerves and some of the internal organs, depending on the position and pressure of the movements involved. In general, the *pressure movements* result in a speeding up of the body's physiology whilst slow, gentle *effleurage* has a soothing effect, calming the nerves and enabling the patient to relax.

When effectively applied, this soothing massage quite often results in sending the patient to sleep.

In this book, no particular method of employing these movements is laid down because it is realised that the movements are used in various combinations for different techniques; in fact most tutors have their own technique and students should be warned against comparing the value of one technique with another except on a physiological basis. It is therefore of great importance that students should understand the physiological effects of the various movements so that they have a clear picture of what they are setting out to achieve, can intelligently interpret the movements which they are taught by their tutors and eventually be in a position to create their own treatment for any unusual condition which may present itself.

It may, therefore, be said that the two most important things to remember about massage are:

(1) The physiological effects of movements—either separately or combined.
(2) When not to massage—this latter being known as the *contra-indications*.

This importance of when not to massage is sometimes used as the standard to differentiate between the amateur and the professional. Quite often, as a result of much practice, the amateur is able to achieve a reasonable standard of physical massage, but what he or she lacks is the knowledge of how and why, and where to apply it, and why and where not to apply it.

Before describing the movements there are several important facts to remember if the student wishes to become a good masseur or masseuse as distinct from a merely accurate one.

(1) It is important to establish a sympathetic relationship with the patient because, as already mentioned, massage has a psychological as well as a physiological effect.

(2) Massage should not hurt the patient except in those therapeutic treatments where the cause is known. Pain or discomfort should always be regarded as a warning signal: either the pressure applied by the therapist is too great for the sensitivity of the patient, or there is a more specific reason for the pain and this should be investigated.

(3) The therapist should stand as close to the couch and the part of the patient being massaged as is reasonably possible. Standing an unnecessary distance away induces back strain and unnecessary fatigue.

(4) Most massage is achieved by using the muscles of the forearm and hand and not by employing the whole of the therapist's body, which again only adds to the fatigue factor.

(5) The patient should be provided with suitable covering—usually in the form of a towelling robe or towel. There are, of course, exceptions but in general it is usually only necessary to uncover the part of the patient's body which is receiving treatment at a particular time and to cover it up again when that part of the body has been treated.

(6) It is essential to maintain a correct, professional attitude towards the patient. See note in the chapter on Professionalism (Chapter 24).

(7) All materials likely to be used during the massage, talc, tissues, etc., should be set out and be close at hand before treatment starts.

(8) The patient's comfort and preferences should be studied as far as is reasonably possible—for example: it is advisable, if possible, to avoid having lighting over the couch in such a way that the patient, in a supine position, stares directly into it.

(9) Never expect a patient to do for themselves something which you could easily do for them; if a limb has to be moved, assist with its movement and, in particular, help the patient on or off the couch.

MOVEMENTS

Just as there are many techniques in massage so there are a variety of movements. But, in practice, they can be condensed into six basic movements, three bearing English names and three with French names. The six basic movements are effleurage, pétrissage, tapotement, kneading, hacking and cupping.

Effleurage

Effleurage is a movement which is mainly done with the flat of the hand, with the fingers close together and, as far as is practical, the tips of the fingers turning upwards so that they avoid protuberances such as the knee. Effleurage *precedes* all other movements because of its relaxing effect, enabling the patient to get used to the therapist's hands, whilst it also *succeeds* all other movements because it increases the blood and lymph flow in and out of the area as well as relaxing the patient.

Effleurage movements are normally made towards the heart because—in addition to the effect of the effleurage on the skin and underlying nerves—it helps to speed up the venous and lymph flow. Effleurage should be reasonably slow and rhythmic, the same speed being employed in both the upward and downward movements with no break or interval between the two. The patient should experience one continuous movement but with a variation of pressure, which is on the upward stroke. This helps to induce in the patient a sense of euphoria or well-being. It is important in effleurage that the whole of the hand should be used and that it should conform to the normal contours of the body. When it is necessary to stimulate an area then quick effleurage is permissible. Stroking is a term which is sometimes applied to this movement.

EFFLEURAGE

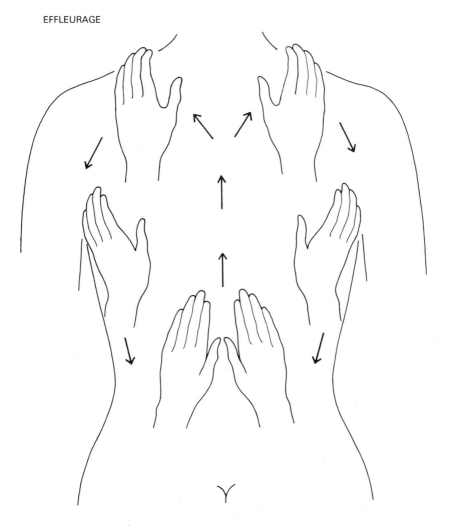

Pétrissage

Pétrissage is normally applied with the balls of the thumb and/or fingers and is applied to soft tissue that has bone immediately underneath it. In this way the balls of the digits are able to squeeze the soft tissue against the bone and so help to eliminate accumulated waste products. It is important in this movement to use the ball of the digit—not the tip—and not to slide over the skin but to securely trap it so that there may be a steady grinding type movement.

Tapotement

These are fine, quick vibratory movements performed with the fingers of one or both hands. They are more often applied to the smaller muscles, for example those of the face, being used for their tonic effect. They are sometimes referred to as vibrations.

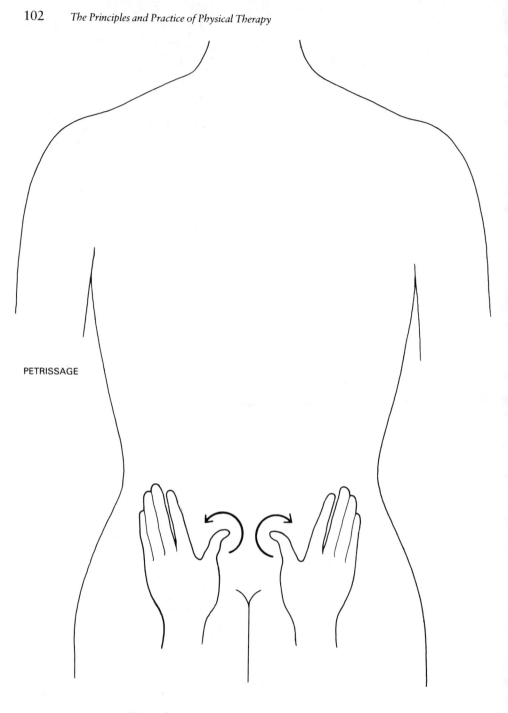

PETRISSAGE

Kneading

Kneading is a very important movement because of its deep effect and because it can be applied to many parts of the body. It is normally used on soft tissue that has no bone immediately underneath it and its action is very similar to that of kneading bread. To knead an area satisfactorily the hands should be dry

(with the application of sufficient talc to the
therapist's hands to achieve this) and the fingers
should be kept straight—that is, in a tension position.
The object is to pick the tissue up and away from the
bone and to roll it back with a squeezing or pressure
action. In this movement it is important not to press
on the thumb but rather to use it as a guide. The
effects of kneading are numerous. It particularly
helps in the elimination of waste products from deep
tissues especially muscular tissue. It assists in the
breaking down of fat, improvement of body
metabolism, muscle contractability and helps the
interchange of tissue fluids. It is also decongestive in
action. *Wringing, picking up* or *lifting up* can be
included under this heading.

Lift

Pull into
palm

Roll over

KNEADING

Hacking

Hacking is achieved with the edge of the hand, with the muscles of the hand in a slightly relaxed condition. If the fingers of the hand are too tense the result is a chopping action rather like a karate chop and this may be painful to the patient. Hacking is used primarily to improve the tone of the muscular tissue and is most generally used on the back, neck and shoulder area although it can be applied to other parts of the body. It has an effect on the larger muscles of the body similar to that of tapotement on small muscles.

Cupping

Cupping is the sixth movement and is a quick movement achieved with the hands in a cupping

CUPPING

position; that is, the finger joints are straight but the hand is bent at the point where the fingers articulate with the palm, and the thumb is brought in closely to create an almost airtight formation. When the hand is brought down on the body, the air which is trapped underneath is expelled, creating a vacuum which, when the hand is quickly taken away, sucks the blood towards the surface and creates a hyperaemia which is very good for the skin, the peripheral nerve endings and subcutaneous tissue. Like hacking, it is most often used on the back, neck and shoulder area but may be used on many other parts of the body. When properly applied it should sound like a horse trotting.

It will be clear that the above movements require a lot of practice before an expert touch is achieved. The following exercises will help to achieve this efficiency more quickly.

Exercise 1   Remove watch or bracelets from wrist and shake the hand quickly but as loosely as possible from the wrist until the whole hand appears like rubber. It is important that this shaking should only be from the wrist and not the whole arm. This should only be done for five to ten seconds at a time although it may be done several times a day. To do it for a longer period of time may only result in the stiffening up of joints instead of the suppleness which it is intended to achieve.

Exercise 2   'Throwing out the fingers': in this exercise the fingers are 'thrown out', that is they are extended and separated as far as possible in order to increase their strength. This should be done for five to ten seconds at a time but several times a day.

Exercise 3   This is an exercise for hacking. The elbows should be tucked closely in to the waist in order to prevent movement of the upper arm. The hacking may be done on a cushion or even on the front of the therapist's thigh. It should take the form of a quick, flicklike movement, the hands operating alternately. To start with, the speed will be slow but this may be gradually increased. If in the speeding up process the hands get out of phase with each other do not try to bring them back into phase but stop and start again. It should eventually be possible to continue this exercise at speed for at least one minute.

Exercise 4   This is an exercise for cupping and is treated in much the same way as the previous exercise—that is the elbows are kept close to the waist and the cupping is done on a cushion or on the front of the therapist's thigh. Other rules are the same as for Exercise 3.

Some Additional Notes on Swedish Massage

Swedish or talc massage is the method or choice for most therapeutic treatments and for slimming treatments. This is because certain movements, particularly pétrissage and kneading, are achieved with much greater effect with talc as opposed to oil when the hands would be inclined to slip. Each movement is executed at least ten times and when done at the correct speed enables a whole talc body massage to be completed in about 50 minutes.

The following is a particular method of approach for a talc body massage. With the patient in a supine position, treatment is begun on the lower part of one leg proceeding to the upper part, then the arm on the same side. Walking around the head of the patient the arm on the opposite side is treated, then the leg, commencing with the lower leg. This brings the therapist into a suitable position to treat the abdomen, waist and lower thorax. The patient then turns over to adopt a prone position and the therapist, who has remained in the same place, treats the leg, then the opposite buttock, then the arm and deltoid area, and walks round the head of the patient to treat the arm on the opposite side, then the leg, followed by the opposite buttock. This places the therapist in a suitable position to undertake treatment of the back, neck and shoulders which concludes a full body massage.

OIL MASSAGE

It is sometimes mistakenly believed that the only difference between oil massage and talc massage is the medium used, but the difference is much more fundamental than this. In talc massage, the therapist's hands are talced so that they may slide easily over the body, whereas in oil massage the patient is oiled so that when pressure is applied the body tends to slide away from the therapist's hands. This means that in oil massage some movements have to be done in the reverse way to talc massage, for example in talc massage of the back, effleurage is applied by the therapist standing parallel to the middle of the patient's body—that is, near the waist area and massaging with an upward pressure over the shoulders and back down again. To achieve this effect with oil, it is necessary to stand at the head of the patient, applying pressure at the waist area and pulling towards the head.

Earlier in this section attention was drawn to the fact that certain movements like kneading are difficult to achieve with oil and that for this reason oil was not the immediate choice for slimming techniques. In addition, there is the fact of the absorption of the oil which many authorities believe provides more calories than it is conceivably possible to counteract by the slimming effect of the massage. Oil massage is, therefore, employed primarily for its relaxation benefits and is used in those conditions where the psychological effects are desired more than the physical ones.

The choice of oil is important—first this should be a thin oil as thick oils tends to become sticky when subjected to the constant friction created by massage. They should be pleasantly but not highly perfumed, so that if used on a female patient, they will not clash with her own personal perfume and when used on a male they will not give the impression of being feminine. A number of good oils are marketed under the generic term *massage oils*. Bearing in mind that oil is primarily used for its psychological effect, the oil should be well presented and it is advisable to pour it into an aesthetically pleasant container rather than the plastic or aluminium bottle in which it is purchased.

Therapists specialising in oil massage should consider the advantages of essential oils treatment. These are aromatic oils chosen for their individual physiological effect and diluted in a suitable vehicle of vegetable origin such as avocado pear oil. A number of these oils are on the market and the manufacturers usually indicate the appropriate uses of the different types. Essential or aromatic oils tend to be expensive but are extremely pleasant oils to use and the effect on the patient usually more than justifies the greater cost of the oil. In other words, these are normally used in costlier treatments—the increased cost being borne by the patient and not the therapist. For more information on the subject of essential oils (aromatherapy) the reader is referred to the writer's book *A Textbook of Holistic Aromatherapy*.

After an oil massage it is very important that the patient should not leave feeling oily. This is normally achieved by wiping the oily areas over with paper tissues impregnated with cologne. When all surface oil has been removed a light dusting of talc is applied.

HOLISTIC MASSAGE

The term holistic is generally interpreted as a treatment related to the whole person—body, mind and spirit. Holistic massage therefore has a variety of movements according to particular schools of thought, but in practice they normally incorporate the use of oil. Movements are slow and of light pressure and involve the whole of the body. Quite often music is used as a background aid.

MECHANICAL MASSAGE

Mechanical massagers fall into two principal types:

(a) Percussors
(b) Gyrators

Percussors operate in a vertical plane; that is their movement is up and down and is approximately equivalent in physiological terms to tapotement or hacking. As the applicators are usually quite small, 2.5–4 cm in diameter, they naturally lend themselves to small areas of operation. Their use is limited to areas requiring tonic treatment and, when using hand-held percussors, to small areas. It must be pointed out that percussors come in a variety of forms, many of which are designed primarily for the home market. They include vibratory cushions, audio-sonic units, vibrating chairs and vibrating or massage belts.

Gyrators, on the other hand, operate in a horizontal plane and may be used to simulate the action of effleurage, pétrissage and kneading. Gyrators are sometimes referred to as *true* mechanical massagers because they approximate most of the actions undertaken by the human hand.

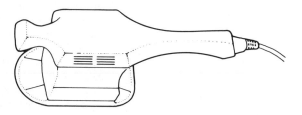

HAND HELD GYRATOR

Gyrators come in hand-held or pedestal form. The effect of both types on the human body is approximately the same—the choice being based on such questions as convenience and impressiveness. Gyrators are widely used in massage at clinic establishments and the reasons for this may be summarised as follows:

(1) They save time—a complete body massage undertaken with a gyrator takes about 15 minutes against 50 minutes if the same areas were covered manually.

(2) Because less time is involved massage becomes a more profitable treatment.

(3) Treatment is achieved with a smaller output of personal energy by the therapist.

(4) The power and depth of penetration of the gyrator means that patients usually experience a deep sense of satisfaction arising from the feeling that their problems are being tackled vigorously.

However, it should be pointed out that whilst complete body massage by means of a gyrator is a time-saving function it lacks some of the aesthetic value achieved when the human hand is used. This makes combined treatments more popular.

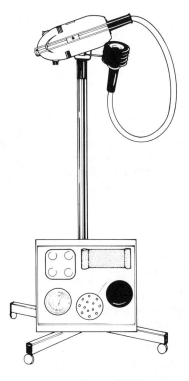

STAND MODEL GYRATOR

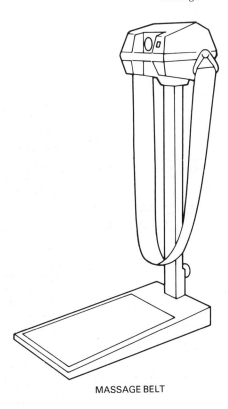

MASSAGE BELT

COMBINED TREATMENTS

Combined treatments are those treatments which involve the use of gyrators on such parts of the body as the arms, legs and buttocks but using the hands on abdomen, waist, lower thorax, back, neck and shoulders. A treatment should take about 25 minutes. In a combined treatment the patient gets the best of both worlds—the power and depth of penetration of the instrument and the soothing, personal touch of the therapist's hand. Most of the movements in the normal Swedish hand massage may be simulated by the instrument so that mechanical massage is really Swedish massage achieved with mechanical aid. Together with the other advantages of combined treatments there is a saving of 50 per cent in the time involved.

One special word of warning—because of their power gyrators should not be used over the abdomen or on the head, breast or genitals.

Most gyrators have a series of alternative heads or applicators. These are usually rubber or plastic in composition and therefore are in no way suitable for use with oil. Oil will not only cause the heads or applicators to perish but will cause a deterioration in the mechanism itself which is usually rubber bushed. Mechanical massagers may only be used with talc.

Another precaution to note is that hand-held models should not be run for more than about 15 minutes continuously—this is because they have powerful motors enclosed in a small area. Despite the fact that they have air circulating fans built into the mechanism, they tend to get warm in use. This is quite normal, but if they are allowed to get hot by continuous running for long periods of time, this will interfere with their efficiency and eventually cause a breakdown in insulation and necessitate repair and perhaps even motor replacement.

CONTRA-INDICATIONS OF MASSAGE

The following list does not claim to be all-enveloping but rather a set of guide lines indicating the areas in which great care has to be exercised.

First and most important of the contra-indications is that therapists should not treat any medical condition except when referred to them by a medically qualified person.

Massage is contra-indicated:

In areas of septic foci (because of the danger of spreading the infection)

In contagious or infectious skin conditions

Over the abdomen during pregnancy (except with medical advice)

Over the abdomen during the first two or three days of menstruation

In cardio-vascular conditions except with medical advice, e.g. thrombosis, phlebitis, angina pectoris, hypertension

In areas of varicose veins

Over areas of unrecognised undulations (lumps and bumps)

Over recent scar tissue

Over areas of unexplained inflammation and pain (these should first be diagnosed by a suitably qualified person)

Any condition being treated by a medically qualified person unless he agrees

Finally in any case of doubt do not hesitate to refer the case to a doctor for his advice.

GLOSSARY

Auto-Infection	communication of disease through one part of the body to another
Contagious	the spread of disease by direct contact with the body of an infected person
Contra-Indications	against, contrary or in opposition to its use
Infectious	spreading of disease through air or by other indirect means
Septic Foci	principal area of sepsis e.g. boils, carbuncles, any condition where pus is present
Traumatic	pertaining to or caused by wound or injury

Chapter 13

Sauna, Steam and other Hydrotherapy Treatments

There is nothing new in the use of thermal baths for the promotion of health. Public and personal hot air and steam baths were very popular in the days of the Roman Empire and the beginning of the use of sauna baths in the northern countries of Europe is lost in antiquity, whilst the hot water baths of the East, particularly Japan, were in existence many years ago. Thermal baths of the past were used for relaxation and socialising as well as for the treatment of disease and it is the purpose of this chapter to show how these age-old ideas are adapted to the 20th century.

Although achieved in different ways the principal effects of heat treatments fall into four categories:

(1) They are used to evaporate moisture from the body. Most of this moisture is obtained from subcutaneous fat which consists of 65–70 per cent water. The amount of water lost from the body in this way can vary from 0.15 litres to as much as 1.5 litres in a single treatment. When combined with dietary control and/or supporting treatments this can result in a reduction in body weight.

(2) By helping the body to perspire they aid elimination of waste products and toxins through the skin. The heat helps to activate the two to three million sweat glands which are in the skin. The liquid exudation from these glands, when subjected to analysis, is found to contain about 10 g of solids—6 g of mineral salts, mainly sodium chloride (common salt), and 4 g of organic substances, mainly urea and urates. If the muscles have been actively working it also contains lactic acid which is the fatigue poison. It will be seen that this exudation is not unlike urine and its discharge through the skin is of considerable help to the kidneys. When sweat baths are used on persons ill from bacterially caused disease, the toxins thus created are rapidly eliminated through the skin—again helping overworked kidneys and reducing the risk of uraemia. The end result of this process of elimination is that the skin itself is thoroughly cleansed and left in a healthier, more elastic state.

(3) They help the body to relax. It has already been indicated in the anatomy section of this book that heat helps the body, and in particular the muscles, to relax and this is aided by the removal, through perspiration, of toxic products. There is also the psychological aspect of being warm, comfortable and looked after by someone else—

in this case, the therapist. The combination of physical and psychological effects result in a deep sense of relaxation.

(4) They prepare the body for subsequent treatment. The success of many physical treatments can be conditioned by the state of the body to receive them. This is particularly noticeable in massage, vacuum suction and those treatments designed to aid relaxation. A warm body is a less tense body, the skin looser and the whole of the body easier to massage as well as giving more pleasure to the patient. Relaxed muscles are also more amenable to faradic treatment and the heat which softens subcutaneous fat makes vacuum suction easier and more efficient.

CONTRA-INDICATIONS TO HEAT TREATMENT

Again these are not the limits of non-treatment but a general guide to the type of conditions which should be avoided.

Firstly no medical condition should be treated except on referral from a medically qualified person

Cardio-vascular conditions in patients—angina pectoris, valvular disease of the heart, history of thrombosis or arteriosclerosis

Abnormally high or low blood pressure

Congestive conditions of the lungs—such respiratory diseases as bronchitis or pulmonary tuberculosis

Skin diseases excepting acne vulgaris

Persons who are under the influence of drugs or alcohol

Any person who is receiving medical treatment —except with a doctor's permission

Within 2–3 hours of a heavy meal

Severe exhaustion

Epilepsy

Persons who have not eaten at all for 5–6 hours, because of the giddiness which may result. (This deficiency can easily be overcome by providing the stomach with some work to do with fruit juices or tea and biscuits)

Diabetes—except with the doctor's permission

During the first 2–3 days of menstruation

During the later stages of pregnancy

HEAT TREATMENT, EQUIPMENT AND METHOD

Steam Baths

Steam baths were originally Roman or Turkish baths—sometimes they were intercommunicating rooms of varying temperatures so that it was possible to progress from cool to hot temperature or vice versa. Though a number of Turkish baths are still in operation the term steam bath is now more usually applied to steam bath cabinets, that is individualised Turkish baths. These may be constructed of metal (usually aluminium), plasticised material or fibreglass. Although they vary in design the basic principles are the same, that is, a single seater cabinet with an aperture for the head and an electrically operated tank or evaporating tray for producing steam. Most cabinets have adjustable seats so that they are capable of accommodating anyone from a small child to a person 2 m (7 feet) tall. Most baths are fitted with rustless water tanks that contain sufficient water to give four to ten baths according to their duration. The heat can usually be controlled by two or three switches. A typical treatment can follow the ensuing pattern:

The water level of the tank is checked to see that there is at least 5 cm of water above the elements; the seat and its front are covered with towelling, the seat itself for hygiene and comfort purposes and the front to prevent steam getting on to the sensitive backs of the legs. A further hygienic touch can be added by putting paper towels on top of the ordinary towels together with a paper towel on that part of the floor on which the feet will rest. A folded towel is put over the aperture at the top of the bath to keep the heat in and the bath is switched on 10–15 minutes before required. Having ascertained that there are no contradictions the therapist takes the patient's towelling gown or towel that she is wrapped in, opens the door and helps the patient into the cabinet as quickly as is reasonably possible to avoid wastage of heat. The towel which was occluding the aperture at the top is now used to wrap around the patient's neck, making sure that all the patient's hair is outside the bath and the timer is set for the required number of minutes. This can vary between 10–25 minutes— with an average of about 20 minutes, rather less for the first one or two treatments. However, these times must not be observed too dogmatically because if the patient feels uncomfortable she should be allowed to come out. Patients' tolerance to heat in a steam bath varies but 50–55 °C may be taken as a reasonable average, that is for those baths fitted with thermometers, otherwise the therapist is dependent on the comfortable feeling that the patient is experiencing—having impressed on the patient that they should feel very comfortably warm—but not too hot. This is a point which should be watched very carefully because quite a lot of people feel that the hotter the bath the more effective it will be and this is not the case. The therapist may add to the sense of luxury of the treatment by occasionally wiping the

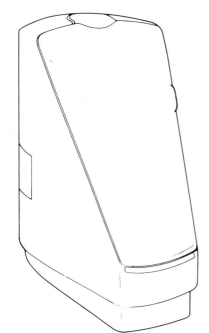

STEAM BATH
CABINET

forehead and/or face of the patient with tissue moistened in cologne or lavender water. At the end of the scheduled time the patient is helped out of the bath and given a brisk rub down to remove the exudation which accumulates on the skin. If the patient is undergoing other treatment he/she is helped on to the couch. If not, it is advisable for him/her to rest in a relaxing chair for at least 15 minutes before getting dressed. If a shower is indicated, this should be warm not cold and taken at the end of the treatment or rest period. Steam baths are not recommended more than every other day and twice a week is a reasonable average except in residential clinics where the patients are under closer supervision.

Sauna Baths

Sauna baths (pronounced sow-na) are usually available in two types: panel sauna and log sauna. Panel saunas are made of outer and inner panels of pine with an air space between. This air space is filled with an insulating material which serves the dual purpose of insulating the bath and thereby saving electricity as well as preventing the heat escaping into the room and altering the room's normal temperature. This is particularly important when the sauna bath is part of the treatment room.

FINNISH
SAUNA

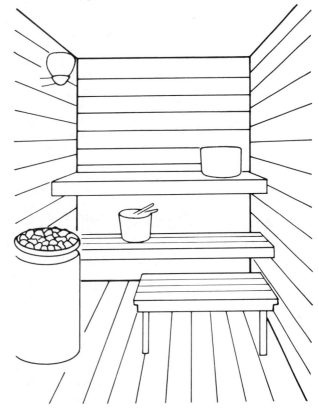

Log saunas are made of solid wood, slightly curved on either side to resemble logs and fitting into each other. They are particularly useful when a bath has to be specially made to fit into an area or alcove. This is not possible with panel saunas which are of pre-determined size. Heating is usually achieved electrically with stoves which have space on top for a quantity of special stones of a non-splintering type.

The smaller sauna baths are capable of being plugged into the normal household supply but the larger ones require a special power cable similar to that used for electric cookers. A qualified electrician should be consulted before commitment to purchasing a sauna bath to ensure that the correct electricity supply is available.

The heaters are controlled by thermostat switches so that it is possible to pre-set to the required temperature. This control should be on the outside of the bath so that it may only be operated by the therapist. Sauna baths usually have a free-hanging thermometer (which should be mounted as near to the top of the bath as possible), a water bucket and ladle. A typical procedure for giving a sauna bath is as follows:

The sauna bath is switched on before it is likely to be required—about 30 minutes in the case of the smaller ones and up to an hour in the larger ones. The seats may be covered with ordinary towelling or paper towelling and the pail filled with water. Although the bath may switch itself off after say 15 minutes this does not mean that it has reached its maximum efficiency. This does not happen until the wood has absorbed sufficient heat to enable it to be re-radiated. Having ascertained that there are no contra-indications, the patient—who is normally just wrapped in a towel—is helped into the bath and advised to sit on the lower level until used to the heat, when he/she progresses to the higher level. Recommended temperatures are between 70–80 °C—the higher figure being for the larger bath where there is a greater volume of air to circulate. Treatment times are similar to those for steam baths, 10–25 minutes—with an average of 20. Some five minutes before the end of the treatment, the therapist should add water to the stones, sprinkling it by means of the ladle as rapidly as possible and quickly closing the door so that the vapour created in this way may be contained. The patient is helped out of the bath at the end of the treatment period and subjected to the same routine as in steam baths. As with steam baths it is very important to avoid overheating the patient because, here too, a lot of people believe that the greater the heat the more they will benefit and this is definitely contrary to the facts.

A recent review of sauna baths in Finland shows

not more than 70 °C to be the common temperature employed.

The practice of alternating periods in the bath with cold showers is to be discouraged. The heat of the bath dilates the capillary blood vessels allowing heat to escape through the skin and reducing the body's internal blood pressure. Subjecting the skin to a cold shower immediately afterwards causes the skin to shrink, closes the pores and pushes up the blood pressure, at the same time keeping in the increased heat. This is physiologically unsound as it subjects the heart to unnecessary strain. Repeating the process several times only adds further to the strain already imposed. In support of the cold shower or cold plunge pool it is sometimes quoted that in its country of origin—Finland—the participants in sauna are frequently rubbed with snow and that, as snow is not available in the slightly warmer climates, the cold shower or plunge is the next best thing. It should here be pointed out that the action of snow on the skin is very different from that of water, snow being used to treat people suffering from frostbite because of its friction qualities whereas cold water would exacerbate the condition. There is, however, very little danger attached to giving sauna baths providing that the correct procedure is adhered to.

Wax Baths

Wax baths are based on paraffin wax; there are several varieties. One example, 'parafango' is volcanic mud from the lakes of Northern Italy mixed into a paraffin wax base. Paraffin wax is a very suitable substance for heat treatment because of its capacity to hold heat and because the human body can tolerate a greater degree of heat in a paraffin wax bath than most other substances. Professional equipment is normally produced in two sizes—the small (or arm) wax bath which holds about 3.2 kg of wax and the large (or foot) bath which holds 20–2 kg of wax.

A paraffin wax bath consists of an outer casing which accommodates the electric heaters and thermostatic control and an inner bath which contains the wax. The outer bath is partially filled with water thus providing more even heat for the wax as well as helping to maintain its heat at a constant temperature. For therapists who may only occasionally be using this form of treatment a very good alternative is to use a domestic double saucepan heated over a gas or electric ring providing care is taken to ensure the wax does not overheat.

Paraffin wax treatments are normally used for small areas, strains, sprains and especially rheumatic conditions. In residential clinics wax treatments are sometimes used more extensively, that is, for whole limbs and occasionally for whole body treatments.

There are four usual methods of application:

(1) The foot or hand is inserted into the bath and allowed to remain there for the period of treatment.

(2) The hand or foot is inserted in the bath and immediately taken out again; the air having a cooling effect on the wax creates a type of glove or sock. This is then wrapped up in towelling or blanketing to keep the heat in and this remains on for the period of the treatment.

(3) The wax is taken out by means of a ladle and spread on to a sheet of plastic to a thickness of about 6 mm. This is then applied much in the same was as a poultice to the parts to be treated and the whole wrapped up in towelling to keep the heat in.

(4) The wax is painted on by means of a brush and the part or, in some cases, the whole body is then wrapped up, first in a rubber or polythene sheet and then in a blanket.

Normal length of treatment is 15–20 minutes. When the treatment is concluded the wax peels off very easily without attaching itself to the hairy surface of the body and *hyperaemia* is revealed.

Foam and Aerated Baths

Whilst these two types of bath are different in effect the mechanism involved is the same. This consists of an air compressor and what is commonly called a 'duck-board'. At one time duckboards were made from a special type of porous wood but now they are invariably made of plastic perforated with hundreds of small holes. The duckboard is placed along the bottom of an ordinary domestic type bath and the electrically operated air compressor forces warm air through the duckboard holes. From here on the two methods differ.

FOAM/AERATED
BATH UNIT

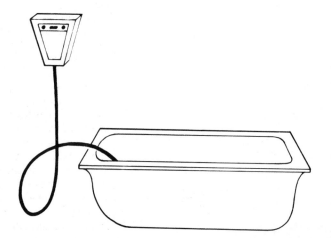

Foam Baths—the duckboard is covered to a depth of about 10 cm of hot water into which is put a quantity of foam extract, usually about 28 g but this depends on concentration. The compressor is then started and continues to run until the foam reaches almost the top of the bath, at which point the patient is helped into a lying position, as in a normal bath, so that only the head is outside the foam. By this time, of course, some of the water which was originally put into the bath has been used in creating the foam, so that the patient is only lying in about 5–7.5 cm of hot water. However, this is sufficient to generate heat in the patient's body and this heat tries to escape in the normal way through the skin. However, the hundreds and thousands of crisp bubbles act as very good insulation and prevent the heat from escaping so that it builds up on the surface of the body. This, in turn, induces more perspiration and the ultimate effect is very similar to that of a steam bath. The normal length of time is 15–20 minutes after which time the patient is taken out, given a warm shower to remove all the clinging foam particles and then given a brisk rub down, followed by treatment or 15 minutes or so of relaxation.

Aerated Baths—here the bath is filled with the normal amount of hot water required for a bath. Into this is put a quantity of seaweed extract, pine extract or other liquid extract of choice; the compressor is then switched on and the patient helped into the bath. By this time the whole of the bath is aerated, being superfused with oxygen, and the patient's body is bombarded by many thousands of little bubbles— the normal length of treatment is about 15 minutes after which the patient is dried and proceeds to either further treatment or relaxation.

HYDROMATIC
BATH

Radiant Heat Baths

Whilst at one time radiant heat baths were manufactured in cabinet form, they are now mainly constructed as tunnel baths. The bath, shaped rather like a tunnel, is made to fit over a standard massage couch and is normally fitted with 12 radiant heat bulbs. At one end of the bath are switches enabling the therapist to control the number of lamps switched on and therefore the amount of heat directing itself on to the patient. The tunnel bath is put over the part of the patient to be treated and the open ends covered in with blankets to maintain a good internal heat. In this way an excellent hyperaemia is produced but comparatively little sweating when compared with the wet heat or vapour bath. Treatment time averages 15—20 minutes but can be as long as half an hour.

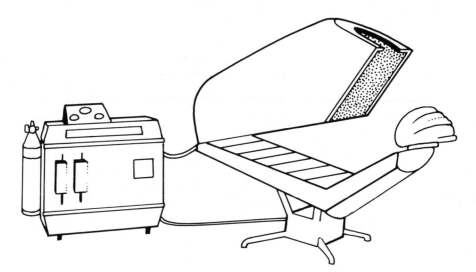

HYDRO/OXYGEN BATH

Reference has already been made to the usual practice of relaxing after steam and sauna baths and then, if a shower is indicated, a warm one should be given at the end of the relaxation period. There are various reasons for this but the two principal ones are that the body continues to perspire for some time, in fact up to 30 minutes, after the conclusion of the steam or sauna bath and a shower would largely stop this process. Secondly, during steam and sauna baths the heart rate usually accelerates as do various other bodily activities, and a suitable period of either treatment or relaxation gives these a chance to return to their normal rate before the patient leaves the clinic and resumes normal activities.

Chapter 14

Vacuum Suction Treatments

INTRODUCTION

Second to massage—vacuum suction must be one of the oldest treatments known to medicine. How far back in history its use goes we do not know but hieroglyphs found on the walls of King Tutankhamen's tomb when it was excavated suggest that the priest/doctors of Egypt used it and during the time of Hippocrates it appears to have been in extensive use.

Reference to an illustration of an early Greek cup which has been found shows that the vacuum was created by operating a plunger at the top of the cup. The Romans—on the other hand—obtained their vacuum in a rather different way. Inside the cup was a wick which was lit and the cup placed over the body. As the oxygen in the cup was used up, the wick went out; the hot air under the cup then cooled, creating a vacuum and sucked the tissue into the cup.

With the renaissance of medicine in the 16th century vacuum suction became a popular form of treatment—the cups by now being manufactured of glass. Bell's cupping jars (19th century) were still being used up to the middle of the 20th century.

Reference to a medical and surgical dictionary published in about 1865—under the term 'cupping'—shows the mode of procedure is first to exhaust the air from one of the glasses by inserting under it a flame from a spirit lamp and then immediately applying it to the body, when the skin is drawn into the exhausted receiver and the vessel is firmly fixed. After remaining on for a few minutes the glass is removed by inserting the nail under the rim and permitting the air to enter—when it instantly drops off.

History records a number of variations in the method especially when practised by country people who often used glass or earthenware vessels with wide mouths, such as jam jars, and heated them up either in hot water or by putting them in an oven. To have them at the right heat to create a good vacuum but not burn the patient obviously required a good deal of skill and experience. Today the vacuum is created by electrically operated pumps and the vacuumatic or inverse pressure measured on a suitable gauge, so that whilst the method is very old the means of applying it is comparatively new and the number of purposes for which it is applied considerably increased.

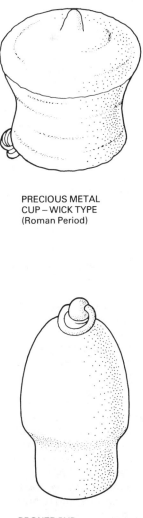

PRECIOUS METAL
CUP – WICK TYPE
(Roman Period)

BRONZE CUP
PISTON TYPE
(Period of
Hippocrates

EQUIPMENT

The equipment consists of an instrument, a series of cups of different sizes (usually 3 or 4 in number) and a plastic tube which connects the cups to the instrument.

Whilst the mode of construction varies with different manufacturers the basic instrument normally consists of the vacuum pump, driven by an electric motor but more usually the pump and motor are an integral unit. The vacuum thus created is measured by a gauge which is normally calibrated in percentages. Scientifically vacuum is measured in inches of mercury so it is important to note that the measurement of these gauges on therapeutic instruments is not in inches of mercury but in percentages. Some instruments are not fitted with gauges but have preset percentage positions. The suction is then applied to the patient via the plastic tube and the cup.

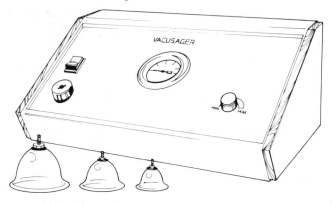

VACUUM
SUCTION INSTRUMENT

Normally these instruments require very little attention except for the exterior parts. The cups need to be kept thoroughly clean and sterile; this is achieved by either keeping them in a sterile cabinet or wiping with a cloth or tissue impregnated with a suitable disinfectant. The connecting tube provides a good lodging place for debris, powder, superfluous oil, etc., sucked off the skin of the patient and this tends to accumulate around the walls of the tube. If cleaned regularly, say once a week, the tube is kept looking clean. If, however, it is allowed to go for a long time before cleaning, the deposits tend to go green and look unpleasant and unhygienic.

Cleaning is effected by immersing the whole tube in a bowl of warm water to which detergent has been added. Allow to soak for about 15 minutes and then run clean water right through the tube from the tap. If the tube has been allowed to go too long without cleaning and the deposit has become encrusted on the tube walls, soak the whole of the tube in a stronger detergent solution for about 30 minutes, then thread a length of string through the tube, tie a knot in one end of the string and pull this slowly through the tube, repeating if necessary several times until the tube is quite clean. Rinse in the way already described. The plastic tube is flexible but not very elastic so, in time, the end of the tube which fits over the cup handle tends to get loose. When this happens the remedy is quite simple—with a pair of scissors you cut about 2 cm off the end of the tube and refit. In time this shortens the tube to the extent that a new piece of tube has to be purchased but it takes a considerable time for this point to be reached.

Most cups are composed of perspex or plexiglass and are, therefore, tough and resilient. However if they should be dropped onto a hard floor and crack or chip they should be immediately taken out of service. Cracked cups are liable to give faulty readings and chipped cups may damage the patient's skin. Some instruments have additional facilities known as static vacuum as distinct from the more usual gliding vacuum. This is for use when the cup is to be kept in one place; the operative or active vacuum (being the greater) sucks the tissue up into the cup but when this is released—as it is by a time mechanism—there is just sufficient vacuum left to hold the cup on to the tissue so that it does not have to be done by hand. In the experience of the writer this is a facility which is not widely used as it would appear that the results normally sought in the physical therapy field are more quickly achieved by the gliding method.

THE USES OF VACUUM SUCTION

First and foremost it increases the lymph and blood flow and, for this reason, the cup is normally moved towards the heart and directed to the nearest lymph node. In the process, that is the picking up of the tissue, including subcutaneous tissue, and moving towards the lymph node, there is a natural tendency to break down the subcutaneous fat and to accelerate its absorption into the lymph vessels, the contents of which are taken to the lymph node. The fat saturated lymph eventually arrives at the thoracic duct or the right lymphatic duct from whence it is passed into the blood stream where it may be used for heat or energy.

Vacuum suction is therefore a useful means of spot slimming but can, obviously, only be successful when combined with a calorie reduced diet otherwise the fat which has been released into the circulatory system becomes superfluous and is redeposited. Vacuum suction has another particular value in physical therapy—that is the reduction of trauma-produced oedema and accelerating the absorption of inter-muscular and subcutaneous infiltrates. It is emphasised that the oedema referred to is the kind caused by athletic and industrial injuries involving sprains, strains, contusions, bursitis and sinovitis and not the oedema that is of organic origin such as renal or cardiac disfunction.

The effects of vacuum suction may therefore be summarised as follows:

Increased blood and lymph flow

Production of hyperaemia

Stimulated metabolism

Improved absorption of intermuscular infiltrates

This list of effects indicates that vacuum suction may reasonably be used for conditions which come within the following categories:

Muscle toning—including post-traumatic and post-natal

Sluggish circulatory troubles (such as chilblains)

Reduction of oedema

Muscular and soft tissue that is overloaded with waste products (such as after prolonged athletic activity, certain forms of fibrositis, etc.)

For accelerating reduction of subcutaneous fat

CONTRA-INDICATIONS OF VACUUM SUCTION

For the treatment of any medical condition until it has been diagnosed by a qualified medical person

Any condition which is being treated by a doctor

Over or very near recent scar tissue

Over varicose veins

On any person who has a history of thrombosis

On an area which has suffered from phlebitis

Over or near parts affected by inflammation or septic foci

Over or near any infectious skin condition

Over the abdomen during the first 2–3 days of menstruation

Over the abdomen during pregnancy

Over the abdomen of anyone prone to hernia

Notes on the Contra-indications

A question which often arises is 'How old must a scar be before the area can be treated?' There can be no hard and fast rule about this but the general guide line is that if the scar is a very small one, as is often seen in modern appendectomy—after about six months, but large scars such as seen in hysterectomies and caesarian section—after about two years, that is unless the patient's doctor or surgeon advises it earlier.

Varicose veins—whilst vacuum suction may not be applied over a vein it may very usefully be applied above the vein—that is between the vein and the heart as the suction effect produced will help to empty the vein and so relieve the sluggish circulation which is normally associated with varicosity.

METHOD OF TREATMENT

The patient should be lying in a position that is comfortable and the muscles relaxed as far as possible. The area to be treated should be covered with a film of oil. There are several excellent oils on the market suitable for the purpose but, if for any reason these are not available, liquid paraffin may be used. Avoid, if possible, such oils as olive oil, sunflower oil, corn oil or castor oil because these tend to become sticky with the constant movement of the cup over the skin and this tends to pull the skin and be uncomfortable to the patient.

If the patient is wearing any underclothes make sure they are protected by paper tissues to prevent them from becoming soiled with the oil. Next, select a cup of suitable size—this should be materially smaller than the part to be treated (as a guide, cup No. 3 for not too fat thighs; cup No. 4 for large ones). Switch on the instrument and allow about 30 seconds for the motor to warm up if it is the first treatment of the day or the room is a bit cold. Then put a thumb completely over the hole in the centre of the cup thus stopping any air flow and with the other hand turn the power output control until the gauge measures the amount of vacuum required. (This action is not necessary when using a preset instrument.) The cup is then put at the most distal part to be treated directly on top of the oil until the soft tissue elevates into the cup. The tissue is then lifted and slowly moved until the cup is over the lymphatic node, care being taken to keep the cup in a level plane during the whole of the movement. When reaching the lymph node the little finger of the hand holding the cup is pulled underneath the cup so as to break the vacuum and the cup returned to the distal area again. This movement is repeated a minimum of six times. The position is then altered by half the width of the cup, and six more slow movements are made. This process is repeated until the whole area has been covered. It is important when breaking the vacuum over the lymphatic node not to tilt the cup as this could result in broken capillaries. The vacuum may only be broken by using the trailing finger method already described or by inserting the tip of the finger of the other hand under the cup. It is also important not to press on a cup during treatment as this could be uncomfortable for the patient.

VACUUMATIC GLIDING TREATMENTS (VACUSAGER)

Arrows indicate direction
of movements to
appropriate lymphatic
nodes

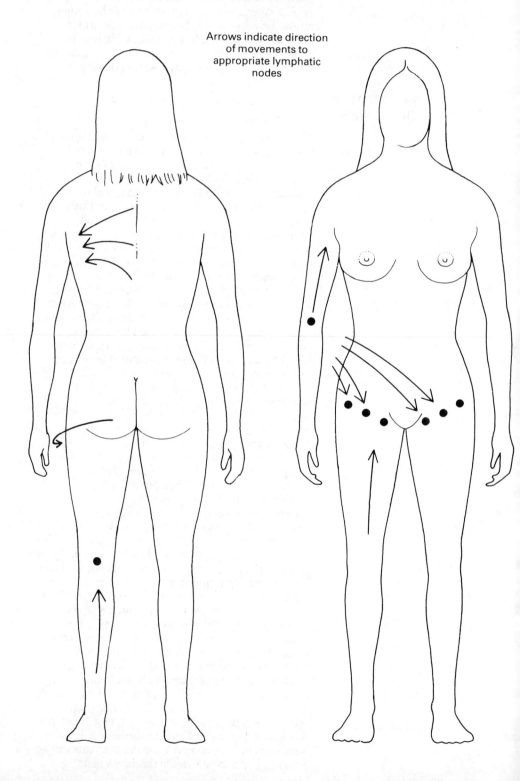

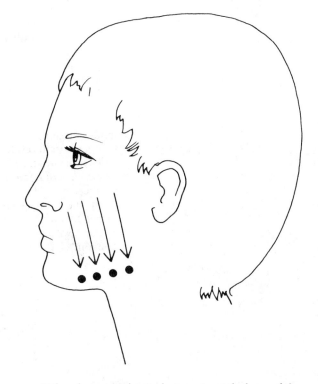

VACUUMATIC GLIDING
TREATMENTS (continued)

When learning this technique it might be useful to remember the following order—cup on, lift, move, break.

At the end of the treatment all traces of oil should be removed by cologne or tonic lotion and then a sprinkling of powder.

In choosing the starting vacuum attention must be paid to the age and condition of the patient. Experience will soon indicate the correct starting vacuum percentages but the following may prove a useful guide until the experience has been achieved:

(1) For young, healthy persons with elastic skin a starting vacuum of 8 per cent.

(2) For middle aged persons or those of delicate disposition 6–7 per cent.

(3) For old people with parchment type skin 5 per cent.

In all these cases the initial percentage should be reduced by 1 per cent when treating the sensitive areas of the body, that is the inner aspects of the thighs and arms, the face or the vicinity of the breasts. This means that where the starting vacuum is 8 per cent these sensitive areas of the patient should be only treated with 7 per cent. Providing the treatment is given more than once a week the vacuum may be increased each time by 1 per cent until a comfortable maximum has been reached which should not normally exceed 15 per cent.

When the patient has been under treatment for some time the number of strokes may be increased from 6 to a maximum of 10. Treatments should be given a minimum of twice a week—once a week not being considered satisfactory because it is not possible to build up the treatments. The ideal is treatment every other day particularly at the beginning of a course. Because vacuum suction is a build-up treatment the patient should be warned not to expect visual results from the first 4–5 treatments, which indicates that the patient should be booked in for a course of not less than ten treatments in the first instance.

One final note—this is not the treatment of choice for patients who are grossly overweight but rather for those who may have accumulated subcutaneous fat in one or two areas.

Chapter 15

Electricity in Treatment

All therapists who use electrical instruments should have a basic understanding of electricity, the precautions necessary when using it, and how to locate and remedy simple faults.

An electric current is a flow of negatively charged particles, *electrons*; the unit of current is the *amp* or *ampere* (sometimes written as A). There are two types of electricity: direct current, flowing in one direction only; and alternating current, which repeatedly changes its direction. Direct current (DC) is supplied by batteries, alternating current (AC) from the mains supply.

An electrical current will only flow between two points if there is a force or *voltage* to drive it. The unit of electrical force is the *volt* (abbreviated as V) named after Volta. The usual voltage for houshold electricity is 240 V although this varies in different countries and cities. It is wise to check the voltage required before purchasing electrical equipment. This information may be found at the electricity meter through which the supply passes from the local Electricity Board.

The *power* required for electrical appliances is measured in *watts* (W in short), named after the inventor of the steam engine. It is equal to the current in amps (A) multiplied by the volage in volts (V). In other words,

Power (in W) = Voltage (in V) × Current (in A)

It is therefore simple to work out the power required to run an electrical appliance from the voltage and current. Equipment constructed for 240 V operation and labelled 10 amp will require 240 × 10 (V × A) W to run, i.e. 2400 W or 2.4 kW (kilowatts).

The current flowing through the appliance can be worked out from the power and voltage, and from this the type of fuse to be fitted to the equipment determined. A 1000 W or 1 kW single-bar electric fire run on the mains supply (240 V) will require 1000/240 A (W/V), i.e. just over 4 A to function. The plug top should therefore be fitted with a 5 A fuse.

Electrical energy is equal to the power of an appliance multiplied by the time for which the appliance is switched on and is measured in *kilowatthours* (kWh). This means that a 1 kW electric fire will use 1 kWh of electricity when switched on for 1 hour. Electricity is charged for according to the number of kilowatthours used by the customer, and the Electricity Boards' name for the kilowatthour is a *unit*. If electricity costs 6 p per unit, it will cost 6 p to run a 1 kW fire for 1 hour.

A single-bar electric fire requiring 2.4 kW to run will use 2.4 kW per hour, i.e. 2.4 kWh, or 2.4 units. At 6 p per unit, this will cost 2.4 × 6 p = 14.4 p an hour to run. Light bulbs which require less power to run than electric fires will cost less to run per hour. A 100 W or 0.1 kW light bulb will use 0.1 kWh and therefore cost 0.6 p per hour to run.

In general, heat-producing equipment (sauna baths, steam baths, radiant heat lamps) is more expensive to run than electronic equipment (faradic units).

Household electricity has two *poles*, live or *positive* and neutral or *negative*. In the heating and power parts of the circuit there is a third wire known as an *earth* wire. These are usually colour coded—most new installations being coded in the following way: the brown wire is live, the blue neutral and the yellow/green earth. In the old installations the live is red, neutral black and earth green. It is absolutely essential that clinic equipment used on a patient should always be connected to an earthed plug, that is a 3 pin plug. It is also important that the apparatus or plug should be suitably fused—that is the value of the fuse should not be much greater than the maximum current (amps) for the equipment.

All therapists should know how to wire up a plug. The attached illustration which is of a 13 amp square pin plug should help. On most plug tops the screws are marked L, N and E which corresponds with the socket into which they are going to be placed so that the brown wire goes to L, the blue wire to N and the green/yellow to E. When the screws are tightened, make sure that the cord grip is screwed up firmly to stop the wires being tugged out and make sure that a cartridge fuse of the right value is inserted before you screw the cover plate back on to the plug top.

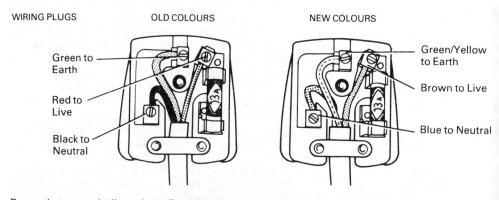

WIRING PLUGS   OLD COLOURS   NEW COLOURS

Green to Earth
Red to Live
Black to Neutral

Green/Yellow to Earth
Brown to Live
Blue to Neutral

Remember: green/yellow wire to Earth terminal (marked E or ⏚); blue wire to Neutral terminal (marked N); brown wire to Live terminal (marked L).

FUSES

It is equally important that therapists should understand the purpose served by fuses.

In simple terms—a fuse is a piece of wire of known resistance. When the current passing through is too great the wire melts. So, for example, if the 1 kW fire (4 amps) to which we have referred earlier, is attached to a circuit which is fused for 3 amps, the fuse will blow (melt) because the current required to run the fire is greater than the fuse wire is able to stand. It can, therefore, easily be seen that the function of fuses is to protect the instrument or equipment so that if anything basically goes wrong with the equipment, the increased current which it draws will blow the fuse. For example, if two wires get crossed, causing a short circuit, instead of burning out the equipment as would be possible, the fuse is blown. It is important when a fuse blows to find out why it has blown because if this is due to a basic fault in the equipment or to wires touching in the lead or plug, renewing the fuse will be of no value since it will simply blow again. If, therefore, a fuse blows a second or third time in quick succession, it is always wise to have the circuit checked by a qualified electrician.

Fuse replacements are in two forms: wire and cartridge. Fused plug tops invariably use cartridge fuses and the fuses built into most modern equipment are in the form of cartidges. The mains fuses—that is those to be found usually near the meter—may be cartridge or wire. The more usual plug-type cartridges are 5 amp and 13 amp and it is always wise to keep a few of these handy in case of emergency. Wire is normally purchased on a card, suitably marked 5, 10 and 15 amp.

When mending a fuse on an instrument, make sure that the plug top is removed from its wall socket. It is not sufficient to just switch off. Before attempting to repair a mains fuse always turn the mains switch to the 'off' position. If the fuseboard is marked in such a way that you can see which plug or set of plugs is served by a particular fuse then it is easy to locate the one that is faulty but it is sometimes necessary to take out a number of fuse holders and inspect the wire to make sure that it is not broken or burnt before finding the correct one. When you have found it, remove the old wire and insert a new piece of wire of the correct amperage. Replace the fuse holder and turn on the mains.

As a guide to the wattage a fuse withstands, and on the basis that the mains electricity is 240 V, a 2 amp fuse will take up to 480 watts, a 5 amp fuse up to 1200 watts, a 10 amp fuse up to 2400 watts and a 13 amp fuse up to 3120 watts. In addition to a small supply of cartridge fuses and fuse wire it is useful to keep a small screwdriver handy.

As a safety precaution:
Equipment should not only be switched off at night but should be unplugged
When fitting adaptors to plug sockets make sure that the socket is not overloaded
Never remove a plug from its socket by pulling on the cable
Do not expose electric cables to excessive heat, for example, do not run them too near a fire
Avoid trailing cables where they may easily be tripped over

DIRECT CURRENT OR BATTERY OPERATED EQUIPMENT

It is well to remember that batteries do not create electricity—they store it and so make it possible for apparatus to be operated independently of a mains supply.

There are two types of batteries in common use: the *throw-away* type, that is the kind which, when its electrical energy has been expended, is of no further value, and the *rechargeable* type. The rechargeable type, though more expensive in the first instance, can be recharged from household current via a charger. Most units of this type are supplied complete with suitable chargers at the time of purchase. Alternatively, sometimes the charger is built into the apparatus. On no account should a rechargeable battery be connected directly to household current without a charger as this would cause the battery to be destroyed. Some battery operated equipment is fitted with a battery indicator but where there is no such indicator on an instrument it is reasonable to assume that the batteries are running down when the power control knob has to be turned up higher to produce the same effect as previously. If for any reason it is intended not to use a battery unit for a considerable time the batteries should be removed. Where there is a choice, batteries of the non-leak type should be used. These are sometimes marked HP batteries and are a little more expensive than standard batteries but longer lasting and their leakproof quality prevents damage to the apparatus.

MEDICAL CURRENTS

The three types of current used in medicine are:

(1) *Faradic*—an induced current named after Faraday who discovered the laws of electromagnetic induction.
(2) *Galvanic*—which is direct current named after Galvani who, using electric batteries first obtained evidence of its effect on frogs.
(3) *Sinusoidal*—or true alternating current of the type we have in normal household electricity. It is so named because its flow represents a sine curve.

The frequency of such alternations is important for the satisfactory running of some electrical equipment and a check should always be made that the equipment has been constructed suitably for the available current. The more usual frequencies for alternating current (AC) are 50 cycles a second, common to the United Kingdom and Europe, and 60 cycles a second common to America. At one time, sinusoidal current was used as a treatment in its own right but the new techniques developed in the manufacture of faradic and galvanic equipment have, to a large extent, caused sinusoidal treatments to be superseded except in certain special categories. This chapter will therefore deal with the two currents popularly in use—faradic and galvanic.

FARADISM

This is used primarily as a muscle exerciser because of the readiness of the muscle fibres to accept this form of stimulation. It is at its most efficient when the pads are placed at the point of origin and the point of insertion of a muscle. This obviates unnecessary wastage of current in surrounding tissue though, because of the conductivity of tissue, it is possible to operate muscles from pads which are placed some distance away from them. This accounts for the variety of pad placement diagrams that are published. All of these work to a greater or lesser extent but those which are based on sound physiological principles will obviously act more efficiently and with a greater economy of current. In general, the two pads or pairs of pads which complete the circuit should be placed at either end of the muscle or group of muscles which are to be activated or—alternatively—over the principal nerve feeding those muscles at one end and the point of attachment of the muscle at the other. For example, a pair of pads placed at either end of the thigh will cause faradic current to flow directly into the muscles whereas pads put on either side of the thigh waste a lot of the current before it is picked up by the motor nerve activating the muscle or group of muscles. When muscles directly cut across the path of other muscles there is bound to be an effect on the second group. For example if treating the abdominis rectus—by putting a pair of pads just above the symphysis pubis and the distal end of the sternum— some of this energy is bound to flow into the abdominis transversalis which runs at right angles. Therefore if another pair of pads is put on the right and left side of the waist it will require proportionately less current than if the position had been reversed—in other words, the first pair of pads to be supplied with faradic energy will require a greater amount of current because of leakage and the second pair a lesser amount of current.

Whilst the output controls of most instruments are calibrated, 0–9 are the more usual ones, it must be remembered that these calibrations only indicate the amount of current which is flowing into the tissue and are no guide to the result you might expect because the amount of current required to move a muscle is conditioned by three factors:

(1) The size of the muscle
(2) The amount of tissue that it has to pass through before reaching the muscle. It should be remembered that subcutaneous fat acts as an insulator rather than a conductor of electrical energy so that a fat person requires considerably more faradic current.
(3) The state of the muscle

Little used muscles, ones lacking in tone or subject to fatigue, require more electrical energy to move them. This may be summarised as size, depth of muscle and tone.

The pads necessary for conducting faradic energy to the muscles come in various forms:

(1) Metal plates—these are usually cut out of pure tin (because of its conductivity factor) and are placed on top of several layers of surgical lint, previously soaked in normal saline solution (salt water). This method is now less used for general treatments because of time and cost.
(2) Semiconductor pads—these are constructed of rubber which, in the process of manufacture, is impregnated with graphite or a similar substance which converts what would otherwise be an insulating material into a semiconducting one. These have the advantage of being easy to apply, easily sterilised and long lasting.
(3) Roller electrodes—these can be very useful especially on smaller muscles such as those of the face, hands and feet.
(4) Handle or disc electrodes which are normally only used when an individual muscle has to be tested or treated.

Faradic Instruments

Hand surged faradic units—of which the Bristow Coil was the most common—have now been almost completely eclipsed by electronic instruments, where the surging is done automatically. There are so many faradic units on the market that it is only possible to give a short description of some of the principal types.

There are small, single or twin output units, usually battery operated, particularly suitable for domiciliary treatments where only small areas have to be treated, for example part of one limb. Multi-output instruments are usually mains operated though not always and come in both transportable and clinic forms. These mains output units are especially suitable for physical therapists who undertake body toning treatments and of these units—the 6-output one is probably the type in most popular use. This has controls for six pairs of pads enabling the whole body to be treated, both legs, both arms, waist and abdomen.

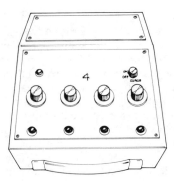

4 OUTPUT (8 PAD)
BATTERY OPERATED
FARADIC UNIT

8 OUTPUT (16 PAD)
FARADIC UNIT
WITH ADDITIONAL
TREATMENT MODES

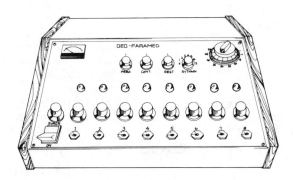

There are individual differences in machines of different manufacture. Some have a fixed surge rate and function at around 50 surges a minute. Most of the medically orientated instruments have a variable surge rate. All have individual power controls for each pair of pads—some have indicator lights which show when a particular circuit is live or in use. Some are completely transistorised in order to make them as small as possible and therefore easily portable. Some are mounted in large cases which may impress the patient, whilst for the therapist seeking to specialise in this type of therapeutic activity, there are instruments with 8 outputs, individual power controls, variable surge rates, indicator lights coloured to match the patient's leads, variable pulse (useful in dealing with different disease conditions), a choice of current rhythms and variable rest times between the contractions.

It will therefore be seen that the therapist has quite

a wide choice of instruments from which to choose—instruments designed for the simplest to the most sophisticated of uses. It should, perhaps, be emphasised that in the multi-output units, not all the outputs have to be used at any one time so, for example, in muscle testing only a single output is needed.

Method of Operation

Having decided which parts of the body are to be treated, the therapist selects the appropriate number of pads with their leads attached. The active surface of the pad (the part to be in contact with the patient) is well moistened with warm, ordinary water. The pads are then applied to the patient, being held in position with rubber or elasticated straps, and the leads then connected to the instrument, making sure that all the power controls are at zero. The instrument is switched on and a suitable surge rate chosen. The power control of the first set of pads is then turned up until there is a visible contraction, then the second pair of pads is dealt with in the same way and so on until all the pads on the patient are producing visible contractions. A timer is set for the length of time that the treatment is intended and when this time has expired, the instrument is turned off (so that all contractions stop simultaneously), each power unit is then turned back to zero and the pads taken off in the reverse order to that in which they were put on. This saves the wires becoming entangled. The pads are then put in a steriliser or wiped clean with a disinfectant-impregnated tissue in readiness for the next treatment.

Surge Rate

This is the rate at which the contractions occur and should be varied according to the condition or age of the person being treated. As a general guide—toning treatment for comparatively healthy, youngish persons can be in the 50–60 surges a minute range. In elderly people this might be reduced to 30–40 a minute. In post-trauma treatment, muscle atony or fatigue, it may be necessary to reduce the surge rate to 20 a minute or even less in some cases.

Time

This, too, is variable according to age and condition of the person treated. A healthy person could have, say, 15 minutes for the first treatment, 20 minutes for the second treatment, 25 minutes for the third and following treatments. Older people might start at 10 minutes and subsequent treatments be increased more gradually; in the case of injuries 5 minutes may be sufficient.

It should be remembered that faradism produces passive exercise and is therefore capable of causing muscle fatigue, particularly in the elderly or those in a low state of health. It should therefore be administered with care, and surge rate and time related.

For example with the surge rate at 50 for 10 minutes the patient receives 500 passive exercises whereas with the surge rate set for 20 only 200 exercises would be involved in the same time. When receiving the first treatment, it is advisable to warn the patient that when the current is turned on the first sensation is a tinging not unlike 'pins and needles' but that as the current is increased this will give way to muscular contractions.

Pad Placement for Faradic Treatments

Broken circles indicate that the pads are on the reverse side of the body.

NORMAL FULL
BODY TREATMENT

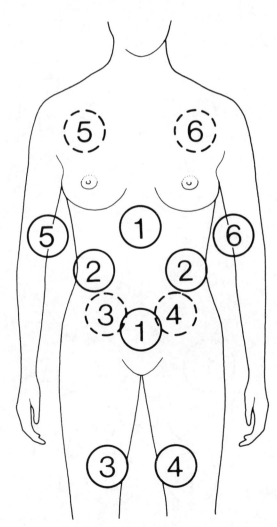

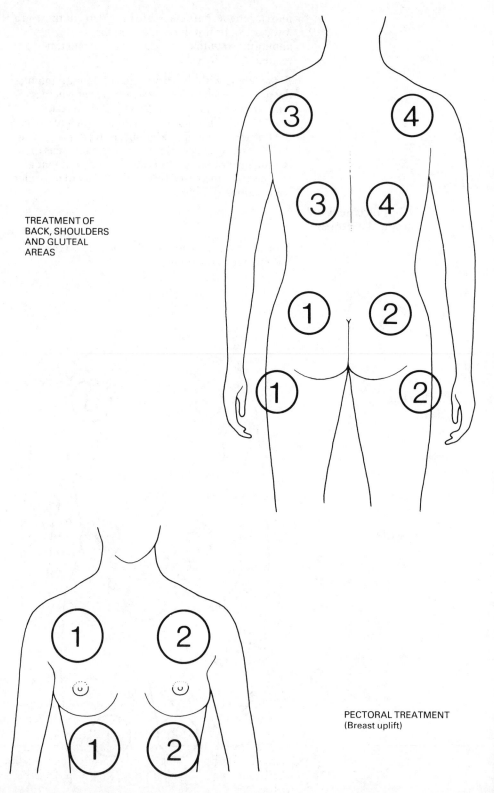

TREATMENT OF
BACK, SHOULDERS
AND GLUTEAL
AREAS

PECTORAL TREATMENT
(Breast uplift)

HIP AND THIGH
TREATMENT

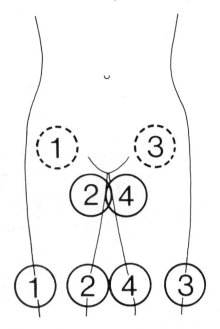

Contra-Indications

With the addition of muscle injury—these are the same as those listed in Chapter 14 under Vacuum Suction Treatment.

Summary of Faradic Treatments

Faradism is used to tone (or shorten) muscles by means of passive exercise. It is not weight reducing in that it does nothing about fat but by increasing the muscle tone it can make a part of the body look smaller.

Surge rate may vary from 20 to 60 per minute.

Length of time may vary from 5–25 minutes with an absolute maximum of 30 minutes, but at no time should this be continued to the point of causing fatigue to the patient.

Current should never be turned up to a point where the contractions appear violent as this can do more harm than good. The contractions should be just easily visible.

GALVANIC TREATMENTS

Galvanic treatments may be divided into two functions, the first—*iontophoresis*—is used with the current as a vehicle to transport substances through the skin into the body and the second—*deincrustation*—has the effect of softening the skin, removing hardened sebum and clearing the skin of the accumulation of oil, traffic pollution and other debris.

The body is composed of cells, and cells, in turn, are composed of atoms. An atom is itself electrically neutral but when it carries a charge it is called an ion—from the Greek meaning 'to wander'. Ions with a positive charge are called *cations* because they are attracted by the cathode or negative pole and ions with a negative charge are called *anions* since they migrate to the anode or positive pole. The unit of measurement used on galvanic instruments is usually the milliamp or one thousandth of an amp. The milliampmeter only registers when there is a resistance between the two poles. When the pads are in position the patient's body acts as the resistance, giving a reading on the meter, but when no 'body' is in the circuit there will be no reaction on the meter even if the output is turned up to its fullest extent.

GALVANIC UNIT

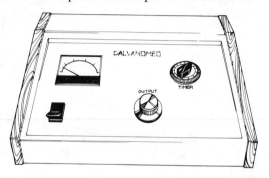

Iontophoresic Treatment

This is a body treatment where the galvanic current is used to carry certain substances such as enzymes into the body for physiological purposes, such as the reduction of fat, e.g. a suitable enzyme having an ingestive effect on the mucopoly saccharides. Because the material so introduced to the body flows to the anode or cathode, according to whether it is negatively or positively charged, it is important to ascertain this fact before commencing the treatment. Most substances supplied for this purpose are clearly marked.

Two metal plates are required, these are usually of soft tin and of a size suitable to the part to be treated, a size of 15×10 cm may be considered average— that is giving 150 cm^2 of electrode surface. In addition two pads of very absorbent material are required and these should be larger than the metal plates so that there is no possibility of the metal touching the skin. The absorbent material may be a number of thicknesses of surgical lint or the spongy type cloth of which there are several proprietary makes on the market. The one pad should be thoroughly soaked with the material to be introduced into the body and the other pad soaked in ordinary water. A typical treatment would be as follows.

First massage the part to be treated so as to produce a hyperaemia. Place the pad soaked in the material to be introduced under the *negative* plate, that is the one connected via the black lead to the black terminal on the instrument and the water-soaked pad under the *positive* electrode, that is the one connected via the red terminal. Turn up the power control (which at this point should be at zero) very gradually until a prickly sensation is experienced by the patient, and then turn up even more slowly until the meter registers 2 mA. Treatment normally lasts 10–15 minutes when the power control is very gradually reduced to zero. The pads are taken off and it is a wise precaution to wash the area of skin that has been under the positive electric plate because in the ionisation process, acid and caustic alkalis are transported from the negative to the positive pole and tend to build up under the positive plate. Neither of the pads may be used again until they have been thoroughly washed. The number of milliamps used for this treatment will vary according to the part treated and the sensitivity of the patient but should be within the range 2–3 mA—this being the amount shown on the milliamp meter.

COMBINED GALVANIC/
HIGH FREQUENCY
UNIT

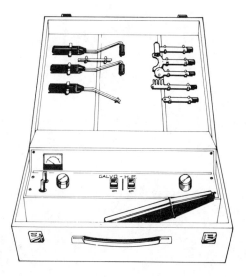

Deincrustation

This is a method normally applied to the face—the material to be used is applied to the face in liquid or gel form. The electrodes, in this case, are usually rollers and these are attached to the negative terminal by means of black leads. The positive electrode is in the form of a rod or bar which is held by the patient to complete the circuit. A current of only a few milliamps is used and the electrodes must be kept constantly on the move—that is, in a rolling action over the face—but must never be allowed to touch each other.

As the aim of deincrustation is to soften and ease impurities out of the skin the current must flow in the opposite direction to that of iontophoresis. This is achieved by putting the switch into the reverse mode. When using an instrument not fitted with a reversing switch all that is necessary is to reverse the leads, i.e. to attach the red lead to the black terminal and vice versa.

Contra-Indications

Galvanic treatment should not be given over varicose veins, pimples or broken skin or any area of septic foci.

If, during treatment, the patient experiences a hot sensation the current should immediately, but slowly, be returned to zero, the pads removed and the area under treatment inspected. To continue treatment under these circumstances can give rise to a galvanic burn.

Chapter 16

Ultraviolet and Infrared Rays

There is often a sense of confusion when a physical therapist is confronted with different types of radiation—*visible light*, *ultraviolet rays*, *infrared rays*, *sun-rays*, *actinic rays*, *radiant heat*.

These are electromagnetic rays or waves. They transfer energy from one point to another without any transfer of matter. They consist of varying electric and magnetic fields which vibrate at a given frequency. Each type of ray has a particular *wavelength* and *frequency*. The different types of radiation are arranged in the electromagnetic spectrum.

Visible light can be split into a band of colours—the *light spectrum*. This effect was first explained by Newton who identified the band of colours red, orange, yellow, green, blue, indigo and violet as separate components of white light.

Visible light has a wavelength of about 1/2000th of a millimetre. The unit of measurement of wavelength in this part of the spectrum is the *Ångström unit* (Å). The Ångström unit is one hundred-millionth of a centimetre (10^{-8} cm, 10^{-10} m). The wavelength of the visible light spectrum ranges from 3900 Å for violet light to 7800 Å for red light.

Ultraviolet rays cannot be seen by the naked eye and have a shorter wavelength than visible light. The ultraviolet band is approximately 250–4000 Å. Ultraviolet lamps used by the physical therapist normally only operate between 2500–3300 Å. *Infrared rays* have a longer wavelength than visible light, they produce heat but cannot be seen.

Frequency is measured in cycles per second or *Hertz*. All electromagnetic waves travel at the same speed so that as the wavelength increases, the frequency of vibration decreases.

The physical therapist is mainly concerned with visible light, ultraviolet rays, infrared rays and waves in the short wave range. Ultraviolet rays cause tanning of the skin but as ultraviolet light is neither visible to the naked eye nor can be felt to be warm, some light from the visible spectrum and infrared range is added to give bluish warm rays known as *sun-rays*.

Infrared rays are invisible heat rays (*black heat*) and can be made visible by the addition of some visible light to give *radiant heat* or heat with light.

The therapeutic value of *actinic rays* was first discovered by a Danish physician, Niels Finsen, at the end of the 19th century. Actinic rays are defined as rays occurring naturally in the sun which produce a chemical reaction, for example, ultraviolet rays, blue and green light from the visible spectrum. This *Finsen*

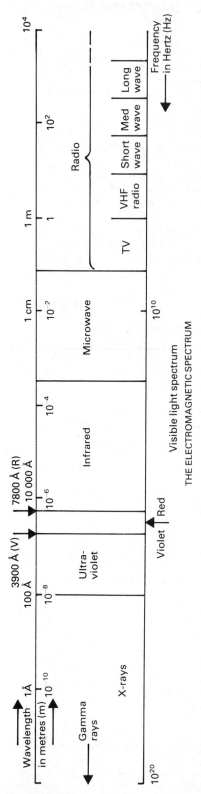

THE ELECTROMAGNETIC SPECTRUM

light was a forerunner of our modern sun-ray lamp. In the early days ultraviolet rays were produced by carbon arc lamps but now most manufacturers employ the high-pressure mercury quartz tube or the longer fluorescent tube which is now used extensively in 'sun-bed' equipment.

The physiological effects of ultraviolet rays vary, depending on wavelength and output. It can generally be said that lamps radiating in the range 2500–2800 Å are *germicidal* in effect while lamps radiating in the range 2800–3300 Å are *cosmetic* in effect. The former range is used extensively in creating a bacteria-free environment, for example in ultraviolet sterilising cabinets or mounted over conveyor belts where it is necessary to have a high degree of sterility. The latter range, that is the 2800–3300 Å, is extensively used in physical therapy because of its effect on the skin, hence the term cosmetic. The two major skin effects of ultra-violet rays are the activation of the chemical *melanin*—the pigment which gives people the healthy bronzed look which so many desire, and the activation of *ergosterol* which produces vitamin D, which, in turn, acts as a calcium catalyst especially for the promotion of healthy bone structure. This is why vitamin D has been known as the anti-rickets vitamin.

Most high pressure mercury vapour tubes produce ultraviolet rays along the spectrum range and to cut out the lower end of this range, which is not normally used for physical therapy treatments, manufacturers employ two methods. In the bulb type generator the quartz tube is encased in a phosphate glass envelope which effectively acts as a filter, cutting out most of the range below 2800 Å but allowing the cosmetic range to come through without alteration. The second method is to fit a sliding filter over the quartz tube. The manufacturers of such lamps claim that the value of a sliding filter is that whilst the filter is over the quartz tube, you have radiation only in the cosmetic range whereas you can, if you wish, slide the filter off the tube so that you have the germicidal range which has certain treatment values.

Manufacturers often refer to the output of their UV products in terms of UVC, UVB and UVA.

UVC is primarily the germicidal range and is eliminated in fluorescent tube units. UVB is in the melanin stimulation range and UVA, which is nearest to the visible light range, darkens the tan started by UVB. Most sunbeds have a little UVB but are mainly UVA.

Ultraviolet rays have one further use in medicine and that is as an aid to diagnosis. When a suitable tube is fitted with a Woods glass filter it will cause certain skin conditions to fluoresce and this method is commonly used in the diagnosis of ringworm.

Summary

Whilst ultraviolet rays may be used for a number of medical treatments the physical therapist is most likely to use them for two purposes—for their tonic effect, produced by the chemical reactions within the body, notably the creation of vitamin D and raising the serum content of calcium and phosphorus—also for their tanning effect which gives the patient a sense of euphoria or well-being.

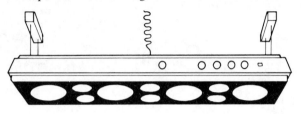

SOLARIUM (Ultra-Violet Rays and Infra Red Rays) Ceiling Fitting

Method of Treatment

The aim of the first treatment is to produce a slight pinking of the skin (*first degree erythemadosis*).

The amount of radiation the patient receives depends on three factors: the power of the lamp, time of exposure and distance of the lamp from the patient.

The intensity of light or radiation depends on the power of the lamp, and as this is likely to vary, the manufacturer's instructions should always be consulted and strictly followed. The time of exposure is critical. If a patient is exposed to the light for 2 minutes, he will receive twice the radiation he would have received in 1 minute.

The set distance between the patient and lamp must always be adhered to. If the distance between the light and the patient is halved, the intensity of light the patient receives increases 4-fold (2^2); similarly if the distance is reduced to one third of the original distance, the intensity increases 9-fold (3^2). (This principle is known as the *inverse square law*.)

The reaction of the skin to radiation differs according to the skin type of the patient and this must always be taken into consideration.

Skin character is normally judged by the natural colour of the hair and is usually divided into three categories:

(1) Average—all the so-called mousey haired people fall into this category.
(2) The natural blonde or natural redhead.
(3) The natural brunette.

Dosage is normally based on the average type; the blondes and redheads requiring less exposure and the brunettes greater exposure.

If the history of the patient indicates unusual reaction to ultraviolet ray exposure then it is possible to do a patch test. An easy way of achieving this is to take a sheet of opaque paper, cut in the paper a line of holes about 4 cm in diameter and 1 cm apart, place this over the inner aspect of the forearm and mount the lamp at the standard distance. Expose the area to the ultraviolet rays for $1\frac{1}{2}$ minutes then cover up the first hole. After a further $\frac{1}{2}$ minute cover up the second hole and the third hole after an additional $\frac{1}{2}$ minute. After a final $\frac{1}{2}$ minute switch off the lamp. The arm should be inspected the following day to see which of the exposure areas most closely resembles a

SOLARIUM
(UVA sun bed)

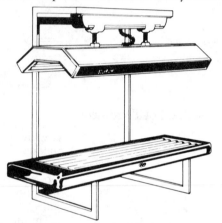

first degree erythema, which will then indicate the exposure time required for the whole body treatment. All parts of the body being treated must be completely free of clothing and the skin free of oil or other skin covering. Before the lamp is switched on the patient must put on goggles of a special type provided for this purpose and such goggles must be worn throughout the treatment, that is, whether the patient is directly facing the light output or not. It is not sufficient to close the eyes or to cover them with pads or material: both methods may allow sufficient ultraviolet rays to penetrate to cause conjunctivitis. The only acceptable precaution is the wearing of these special occlusive goggles the whole of the time the lamp is on. It is also advisable for the therapist to wear protective goggles because, although not directly under the light, she/he may be subjected to a certain amount of scatter radiation which will build up when there are a number of treatments during the course of the day.

The following is a typical treatment for ultraviolet lamps of the bulb type or those fitted with filters:

The patient is lying on the couch in a supine position and with protective goggles in place. The ultraviolet lamp should be exactly 60 cm from the patient, the distance measured between the lamp and the part of the patient nearest to it. In the female patient this is likely to be the breast area whereas in an obese man it would be the abdomen. The patient of average skin type should be exposed for exactly $2\frac{1}{2}$ minutes and then turned over into the prone position and exposed for a further $2\frac{1}{2}$ minutes when the lamp is switched off and the goggles removed. If the patient is a natural blonde or redhead the treatment time should be reduced to 2 minutes whilst, for the natural brunette, it should be increased to 3 minutes either side. Providing the treatment is given at least twice a week, each subsequent treatment may be increased by half a minute either side and treatment may be continued until a maximum of ten minutes either side is reached. When this point is reached treatment is either discontinued or, if the patient wants to keep up the achieved tan, radiation on the basis of once a week at the maximum dosage of ten minutes either side may be given. The patient should be told that there is not an immediate reaction to ultraviolet rays but that such reaction usually occurs between one to eight hours after treatment when the slight pinking should become visible. This is sometimes accompanied by an itching sensation due to the drying action of ultraviolet rays but this can, to a large extent, be guarded against by the use of a suitable oil or moisturising cream after treatment.

Contra-Indications

All medical conditions except when under the direction of a medically qualified person
Congestive conditions of the lungs—for example bronchitis
Advanced cardio-vascular troubles—for example angina pectoris
Arterioscelerosis
Photosensitive skins, that is those skins which have an abnormal reaction when exposed to normal sunlight
Vitiligo—a condition in which patches of the skin are devoid of pigmentation
Skin diseases except under medical direction (skin cancer is itself associated with exposure to ultraviolet rays)

In patients with kidney or liver complaints over exposure can produce headaches, vomiting, nausea, faintness and insomnia.

Pigmentation of the skin to the extent that we refer to it as 'sun-tanned' is the body's natural protection against the admission of too great a quantity of ultra-violet rays so that the more tanned a body is—the fewer ultraviolet rays are able to penetrate. It is worth noting however that this pigmentation factor can be affected by drugs, some of which are widely used in medical treatment. If, therefore, the patient presents unusual reactions to ultraviolet ray therapy their current medical habits should be checked in consultation with their doctor. Certain drugs and antibiotics sensitize the skin. If in doubt check with the client's doctor.

INFRARED

It has already been mentioned that radiant heat is infrared rays plus some of the visible part of the spectrum. The physiological effects of black heat and radiant heat are almost identical but there are certain practical advantages to be found in radiant heat which account for it being the more popular form of treatment.

These advantages may be summarised as follows:

(1) Radiant heat generators normally reach their peak output 30 seconds after switching on whereas infrared generators generally require up to 10 minutes to reach peak effect.

(2) Radiant heat lamps normally have a built-in reflector system which projects the waves from the lamp in a more or less parallel beam resulting in fairly evenly dispersed heating whereas infrared generators depend on being mounted in a parabolic reflector and these tend to concentrate the rays in certain areas known as 'hot spots' which means that the heating is rather uneven.

(3) Thirdly, there is a certain psychological value to be obtained from the warm red glow which is given out by a radiant heat lamp as compared with the absence of light from infrared generators.

Infrared rays have often been described as anti-inflammatory rays and this is indicative of their main usage. It is generally agreed that the physiological effects of infrared radiation fall into three categories:

(1) Hyperaemia producing
(2) Relief of pain
(3) Tissue relaxation

Hyperaemia

In all local heating processes hyperaemia is an essential factor including, as it does, the dilation of local tissue blood and lymph vessels and an increased flow of blood, which in turn brings in oxygen and nutriment. Congestion is relieved and the increased circulation promotes tissue repair.

Relief of Pain

This is fostered by the analgesic action of the rays on nerve terminals and by the relief of spasm and cramp.

Tissue Relaxation

The increased arterial flow due to the local application of heat causes the walls of the smaller arteries to relax and the vessels dilate whilst the increased venous flow carries away a large quantity of waste products and toxins.

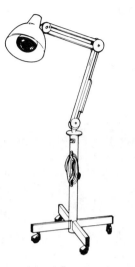

SINGLE-HEADED TREATMENT LAMP
(ultraviolet rays and infrared)

As distinct from ultraviolet ray treatment—the duration involved in infrared treatment is not critical. It is generally agreed that 20–30 minutes is a reasonable period for treatment time but this can be considerably exceeded without any deleterious effect. The correct distance from the lamp to the body is normally determined by the part under treatment being warm but not hot. If the treatment feels hot to the patient the lamp should be moved further away. The patient should be warned of the dangers of tolerating greater heat in the mistaken belief that this will improve the value of the treatment. It may only result in a burn.

Infrared treatments are normally given for traumatic conditions such as sprains and strains and affections of joints and tendons, rheumatism and contusions. Even when its effect is not curative the heat often has a soothing effect which is, in itself, often an aid to healing.

Method of Treatment

A typical radiant heat treatment would be as follows:

Uncover the part to be treated, removing all bandages, plaster, etc., and make sure that the part is free of oil or embrocation. Switch the lamp on about 30 seconds before commencing treatment and position the bulb so that it is directly over the part to be treated and at such a distance that the part is comfortably warm but not hot. Treat for 25 minutes once or twice a day as required. Make sure that the treated part is not exposed to cold or draught after the treatment.

Contra-Indications

Particular care must be exercised in treating diabetic patients because of their lessened sensitivity to heat.

Contact lenses must be removed before any treatment is given to the face because they act rather like a magnifying glass in intensifying the heat.

Chapter 17

Exercises

Exercises are performed in three ways: *passive, active* and *restive*. We have already seen an example of passive exercise in the section on faradism—that is exercise which is mechanically induced and receives neither help nor resistance from the patient.

Another example is to be found in immediate post trauma treatment when the therapist takes the limb and moves it in such a way as to exercise the muscles involved but again without any help from the patient.

Active exercise—this is the second stage of post traumatic treatment and it is the point at which the patient is able to move the muscles himself without any help from the therapist. Another example is to be found in a free cycling movement, that is, pedalling, but without any resistance.

Resistive exercise—this is the third stage in post traumatic treatment and this point is reached when the patient is able to accept a resistance against his/her active exercise. An example of this is to be found when the therapist holds the limb in such a way as to allow movement but only against such resistance as he/she feels it necessary to exert and this is gradually increased as the injured part improves. Another example of this is found in a static bicycle which is fitted with a weighted flywheel or a resistance block so that the patient has to pedal against a load.

The Purpose of Exercise

All exercise is aimed at increasing the fitness of a part of the body, or the whole, and it achieves this by strengthening muscles, improving body metabolism and increasing the efficiency of the blood transport organs. Exercise may be undertaken without any external aids, or it is possible to employ various mechanical devices to assist the patient. Whichever method is used it is essential that these exercises should have rhythm and continuity—ten minutes exercise each day is very much better than sixty minutes exercise once a week.

It is not the purpose of this chapter to deal extensively with self-activated exercise as there are many excellent books which deal with this subject.

The illustrations indicate the parts of the body which are primarily affected by these basic exercises and it is hoped that the information will be sufficient to give the physical therapist a basis on which to build.

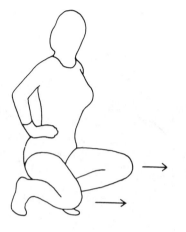

Fig. 1: DUCK WADDLE
(to trim buttocks and hips)

Fig. 2: CYCLING
(for hips and
abdomen)

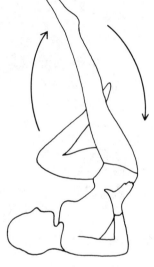

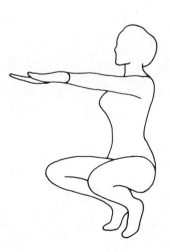

Fig. 3: KNEES BEND
(for thighs and
ankles)

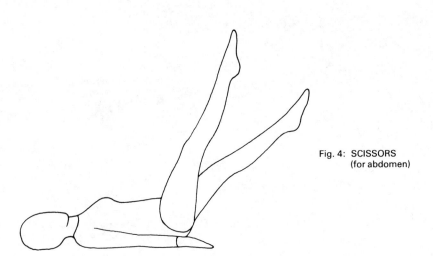

Fig. 4: SCISSORS
        (for abdomen)

Fig. 5: PUSH AND PULL
        – Legs Moving
        Alternately (for
        abdomen)

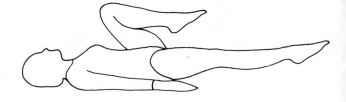

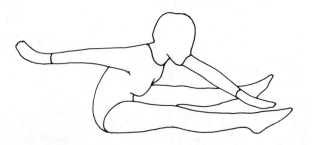

Fig. 6: THE TWIST
        (for waist)

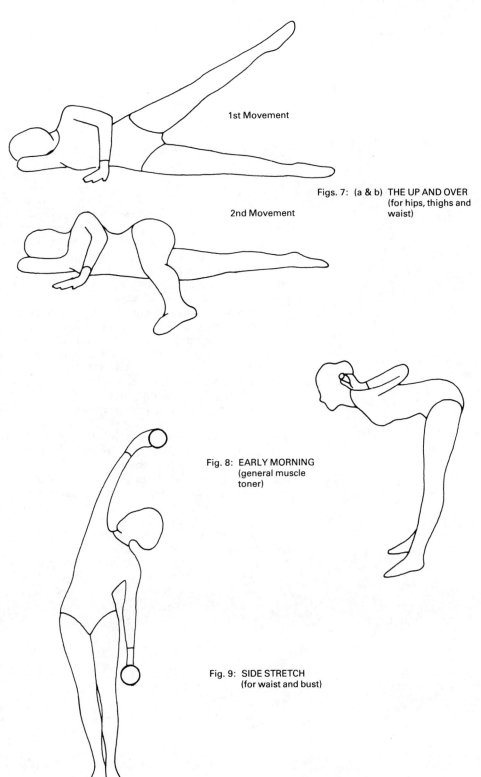

1st Movement

2nd Movement

Figs. 7: (a & b) THE UP AND OVER
(for hips, thighs and
waist)

Fig. 8: EARLY MORNING
(general muscle
toner)

Fig. 9: SIDE STRETCH
(for waist and bust)

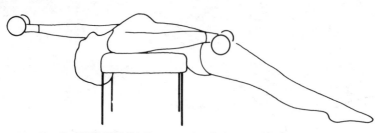

Fig. 10: THE WINDMILL (for contouring the bust and hips)

Mechanical Exercisers

There are many aids to active exercise varying from a simple skipping rope to complex spring mechanisms but a physical therapist is more likely to be interested in *ergometers*, that is, aids which have been designed for resistive exercise and in such a way that the amount of resistance can be measured. The two most popular forms of ergometer exercisers are the ergometric bicycle and the ergo-rowing exerciser. The bicycle type is obviously more useful for the legs whereas the rowing exerciser is especially useful for muscles involving the abdomen, back, shoulders and arms—but with useful leg exercises as well.

The resistance is usually measured in kilogrammes or pounds and the more sophisticated bicycle ergometers are fitted with milometers and speedometers whilst the rowing exerciser may be fitted with a movement counter. It will, therefore, be seen that with an ergometer it is possible to plan a complete programme of exercises, varying the speed, time and resistance. Whilst originally designed for muscle re-education and strengthening, ergometers are now increasingly used for keeping people healthy and, with this particularly in mind, the manufacturers usually supply with the ergometer special programmes and advice on how their particular machine may be used in order to obtain maximum results.

ROWING
MACHINE

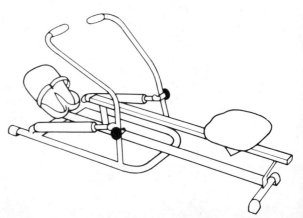

EXERCISE BICYCLE

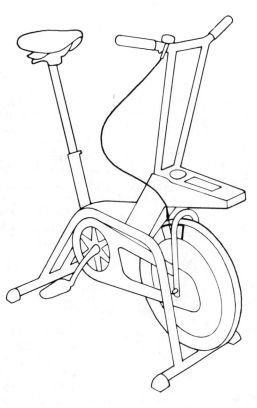

JOGGING EXERCISER

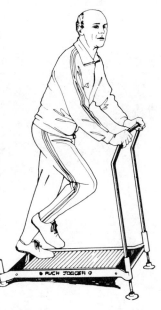

Chapter 18

Other Forms of Treatment

In addition to the treatments which have been described in some detail in the preceding chapters there are a number of other electrical type treatments about which the physical therapist should know enough to understand their function and how they differ from each other. This chapter, therefore, confines itself to an explanation of the type of equipment used for these treatments and the physiological effects which they achieve.

It does not come within the purview of a book of this kind to detail how these many and varied treatments may be applied. For this purpose many excellent books have been published and the therapist is referred to these for much more detailed information. Whilst, therefore, this chapter may not be regarded as a treatment chapter in the ordinary sense of the word it is hoped that it will complete the picture by giving the therapist a clear indication of the alternative forms of treatment available.

HIGH FREQUENCY

The term 'high frequency', as applied to the apparatus usually known by this name, is in itself misleading. When they first came into use the currents *were* high frequency but they have now been superseded by much faster currents which really make them *medium frequency* currents. The dividing line between low and high frequency currents is, in medicine, considered to be 100 000 cycles per second, because beyond this frequency no tetanus sets in.

The original work in this field was done by Nicolai Tesla who gave his name to the Tesla Coil and this field was further explored and developed by the French physiologist, Jean d'Arsonval, who died in 1940 at the age of 89. The work to which we are referring was carried out mainly at the end of the 19th and beginning of the 20th century.

Originally, the equipment involved was large and cumbersome and the patient sat inside a specially constructed spiral cage. Now the equipment is comparatively small and the current applied by means of a hand-held applicator. Many claims were made for d'Arsonval's therapy but it is generally agreed that these may now be limited to a dermal effect. This falls into four categories:

(1) *Effluvation*—that is, contact treatment with one of the glass electrodes, used especially in those skin conditions where raising the skin temperature is of value.

(2) *Spark treatment*—is when a glass electrode is

held a very short distance away from the skin, sufficient for a spark gap to be created between the electrode and the patient. In this treatment the electrode is continuously moved over the area and in this way provides an alternative method of producing a gentle warmth in the skin under treatment.

(3) *Saturation*—so named because the patient becomes saturated with current. In this treatment the patient holds a metal bar or saturator after it has been inserted in the applicator holder and the therapist treats, with hands or fingers, a distant part of the body such as the face, the sensation being on the skin immediately under the therapist's fingers.

(4) *Fulguration*—this is a form of cauterising by using a special applicator. It is sometimes employed on skin conditions such as warts or verrucae.

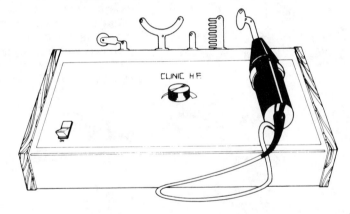

HIGH FREQUENCY
(clinical model)

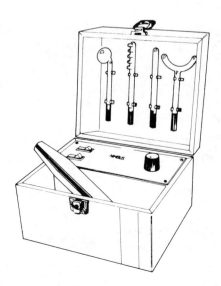

HIGH FREQUENCY
(portable model)

It is important to note that whilst the patient is undergoing treatment he/she must not touch the machine in any way nor put his/her hand on any metallic objects such as metal struts of the treatment couch or chair. In both effluvation and spark treatment it is usual to apply a thin coating of oil to the skin before treatment.

Most of the glass electrodes emit a bluish violet light whilst in use, which has led to them being sometimes referred to as violet rays. They are not to be confused with ultraviolet rays because there is absolutely no connection.

DIATHERMY

Diathermic epilation is the method used for the removal of superfluous hair from the face or other parts of the body and the treatment is often known by its alternative name of *electrology*, because originally hair was removed by inserting a galvanic needle into the hair follicle. Whilst the galvanic method is still being used in obstinate cases, the more usual method is to use a short wave diathermy instrument with a frequency of about 27 000 000 cycles a second, that is, 27 megahertz. A cold light magnifier is useful for studying the hair.

Clinical model

DIATHERMIC
EPILATION
UNITS

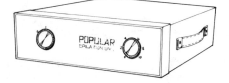

Portable model

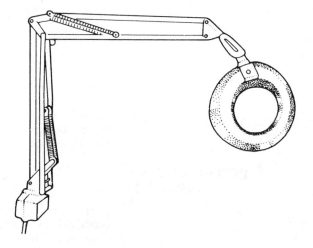

COLD LIGHT
MAGNIFIER

SHORT WAVE

When applied to the body these short waves provide heating in depth which makes them suitable for the treatment of joints and muscular tissue in particular. Application is normally in one of two forms—by rubber condenser pads which are placed on either side of the joint or part to be treated, with a thick separator placed directly between the pad and the patient's skin. These pliable electrodes may be moulded to fit the contours of the body and are held in place with rubber straps.

The second method of application is by means of air space electrodes. These are of rigid construction and again are normally placed on either side of the part to be treated leaving, in this instance, an air space between them and the patient's body. Treatment time varies with the conditions to be treated but an average of fifteen minutes may be considered normal. It is very important when using short wave currents to make certain that no metallic objects appear within the field of treatment. This includes metallic jewellery or supports on the *outside* of the body and metal plates or pins *within* the body. The patient's leads, that is the cables which connect the instrument to the electrodes, must never be allowed to cross each other nor make contact with any metal object such as the instrument itself or the metal supports of a trolley.

MICROWAVE

Microwave—this is a mono-polar treatment, that is there is only one output head, and the electromagnetic oscillations are very much shorter than those of short waves, corresponding to a frequency of about 2450 megahertz. In short wave treatment a good deal of the heat that is generated occurs in the subcutaneous fat tissue. This can be as much as ten times greater than that of the deep muscular tissue. With the very much shorter waves of microwave considerably less heat is created in subcutaneous fatty tissue and therefore proportionately more in the muscular tissue. Treatment times are approximately the same as for short wave and similar physiological conditions are treated but many therapists maintain that microwaves are easier to apply. As with short wave, metal must not appear within the field of treatment.

INTERFERENTIAL CURRENTS

Interferential current is really two frequencies slightly out of phase with each other, for example, if a frequency of 4000 megahertz has another frequency of 3900 megahertz superimposed on it, this gives a beat rhythm of 100 cycles—that is, the difference between the two. The manufacturers of this type of equipment claim that very low frequency has a stimulating effect on tissue whilst, due to a decrease in skin resistance, higher intensities are possible. Beat frequencies of 0–100 cycles are the normal pattern of manufacture and reference books on this subject suggest the selection of different frequencies for a variety of soft tissue conditions.

Chapter 19

First-aid

This chapter is not intended to deal in detail with such an extensive subject, but rather to indicate guidelines for the treatment of some of the more common conditions met with in clinics and leisure centres. For further study the reader is referred to the *First-aid Manual* (the authorised publication of the St John Ambulance, St Andrew's Association and the British Red Cross Society).

FAINTING

This is a brief loss of consciousness created by a temporary reduction of blood flow to the brain. It has a variety of causes including exhaustion, lack of food, pain and emotional upset.

Treatment: Sit the patient down putting the head between knees and advise taking deep breaths. Loosen tight clothing particularly at the neck, chest and waist.

BRUISING

Raise the injured part to a position the patient finds comfortable and apply cold compresses.

SHOCK

This is sometimes accompanied by cold clammy skin and/or sweating.

Treatment: Be firm and positive with the patient and especially reassuring. Lay the patient down in a supine position with the head low on one side. Cover with a blanket, keep the patient warm and summon medical assistance.

MINOR BURNS AND SCALDS

Place the injured part under slow-running cold water (or, if this is not available, immerse in a container of cold water) for ten minutes or such time as the pain persists. Remove rings, bracelets etc. because of the risk of swelling and cover with a sterile (non-fluffy) dressing.

BLEEDING

Most haemorrhages can be controlled with a pressure pad or with the thumb and fingers. In the case of the former a sterile pad should be used and bandaged firmly in place. When the bleeding is from a varicose vein (usually a leg) lay the patient on his or her back, remove any constricting clothes and elevate the leg on a chair or suitable object. Arrange for the patient to be taken to hospital.

HEAT EXHAUSTION

The patient may have a headache and feel very tired and dizzy. The breathing may be fast and the pulse rapid. Cramp in the lower limbs is not uncommon.

Treatment: Lay the patient down in a cool place, provide sips of cold water and seek medical help.

CHOKING

If the patient is conscious, coughing to dislodge the offending object may be all that is needed. If necessary this may be followed by a jolt to the back (back slapping). If these fail then apply an abdominal thrust. This should be left until last because of the danger of injuring the internal organs. The abdominal thrust is achieved by putting one arm around the patient with the clenched fist thumb inwards between the navel and distal sternum. Grasp the fist with the other hand and pull towards you with a quick inward and upward thrust from the elbows. Repeat up to four times.

FRACTURES

In the case of a fracture of the clavicle or a shoulder dislocation, support the arm in a diagonal position with a sling, scarf or other suitable material. With other fractures, immobilize and support in the position found. Do not attempt to straighten a limb where a fracture is suspected. Arrange for the patient to be taken to hospital.

CARDIAC ARREST

(This treatment also applies to other conditions where breathing has stopped.) Place the patient in a supine position with the head tilted back. Make sure that the airway is clear of loose dentures etc. To stop the tongue obstructing the airway, the patient's neck needs to be extended. To do this, place one hand under the neck and the other on the forehead. The latter pushes the head back when the neck hand is lifted.

Leaving one hand under the neck use the other one to pinch the nose. Place your lips over the patient's mouth making a complete seal and exhale into the patient at least four times in quick succession, then repeat if necessary.

It is advisable to practise this method so as to be efficient should the occasion arise. Contact one of the aforementioned organisations or other training agencies and join one of their classes on artificial ventilation.

ACCIDENT BOOK

All accidents however small should be recorded
giving as much detail as possible including: name and
address of casualty, nature of accident as observed at
the time, time of accident, first-aid treatment given,
names and addresses of any witnesses.

Part III

Specialised Aspects of Physical Therapy

Chapter 20

Sports Therapy

SPORTS-TYPE INJURIES AND THEIR TREATMENT

Athletics and leisure-type pursuits which involve vigorous exercise have been with us for a very long time. Recently they have taken on a new importance, partly because of the increased leisure which is available to most people and partly because of the way in which they have been linked to health in general and prevention of certain conditions of ill-health, in particular obesity and heart disease. As more people become involved in this type of activity there is bound to be an increased number of injuries and it is estimated that up to ten per cent of casualties treated in hospital fall into the category of sports-type. These injuries are not necessarily caused by sport but they do, however, fall into a particular category. It will be obvious that an ankle sprained by falling down stairs needs the same treatment as an ankle sprained on the football field.

This chapter is therefore aimed at giving guidance as to the initial or first-aid treatment of such injuries, it being generally agreed that correct treatment in the early stages can often prevent unnecessary complications and in this way considerably reduce the rehabilitation period.

Many injuries should, of course, have specialist treatment. Even with the slightest suspicion there should be no hesitation whatsoever in sending such patients to the nearest hospital, or, alternatively, to their own doctor who may be able to direct them to a specialist in sports medicine.

Sports medicine in itself is by no means a new speciality. At the time of the Greek empire much emphasis was placed on the fitness of young men and those who excelled at athletics were treated almost as young Gods. Subsequently, special provision was made for treatment of injuries received in such sporting activities. Hypocrates had a gymnasium which was roughly equivalent to a physiotherapy department of a modern hospital. Some of the treatments, notably massage and exercise, do not differ materially from those employed today. It is believed that the first doctor to receive an official appointment in sports medicine was Galen, who was appointed team physician to the Perganum Gladiators in AD 157.

General Information

In a chapter devoted to sports therapy it is not inappropriate to point out that prevention of sports-type injuries is better than cure and many can be prevented by following a few simple rules. First amongst these is the importance of warming-up before engaging in the sports in question. This involves stretching all muscle groups with exercises like toe touching, gentle jogging, spot walking, etc. The body is like a motor car—it performs better when warmed. This applies not only to participation in professional athletics but in such pleasure pursuits as tennis.

Next in importance comes the warm-down, sometimes referred to as the cool-down. This enables the muscles to revert gradually to their normal function and it assists in the dispersion from the muscle of waste material, in particular urea and lactic acid, built up during the active phase.

Next on the list must come suitable clothing. Most sports have clothes which are particularly designed for them, emphasis being placed on comfort and freedom of movement. Inappropriate clothing can give rise to friction and such conditions as jogger's or runner's nipple can be prevented in the female by the use of properly designed sports bras and in the male by covering the area with a plaster.

Footwear is, of course, very important and the fitting of shoes or boots should be undertaken with a great deal of care.

In the consideration of preventative measures, rest is of major concern. It is asking for trouble to expect the body to perform well when it is tired and it is in this phase that a large number of injuries take place.

First-aid

You are referred to chapter 19, which deals in a general way with this subject, the following problems being particularly associated with sport.

Blisters—particularly on the feet, can often be prevented by coating the feet with petroleum jelly (vaseline) or by wearing two pairs of socks. These, of course, should not be of the nylon variety because nylon is non-absorbent. However, when a blister has formed and it is found necessary to prick it, this should be done with a pin or needle which has been heated by a match or candle until it is red hot and then cooled under the tap. After pricking, the blister should be covered immediately with a sterile dressing.

Abrasions—are, of course, a common occurrence and should be treated by washing the area gently with diluted Dettol, TCP or a similar solution, making sure that no particles of dirt remain, because when healing takes place these can leave tattoo-type marks.

Cramp—is another problem which is often encountered. This is an involuntary shortening of a muscle quite often associated with excessive sweating causing a consequent loss of salt (sodium), or with chilling, for example in swimming. Treatment involves stretching the muscle and firm massage.

Finally, under this heading, no food or drink of any kind should be given to seriously injured persons because this would delay the effect of anaesthetics in subsequent treatments.

It is worth noting that the use of alcohol (brandy and the like) is not to be encouraged as alcohol dilates the surface blood vessels causing consequent loss of heat, so that whilst the patient may feel warmer the body is getting colder.

Therapist's sports kit

Some therapists are content with throwing a few useful items into a bag and hoping for the best, the usual result being that the one thing they need is missing. A little careful thought can avoid this contingency. The following list is, therefore, given purely as a guide to which may be added such items as the particular sport determines:
Scissors
Crepe bandage (two-inch)
One- and two-inch gauze bandage
Triangular bandage
Cotton wool
Sterile gauze pads
Roll of adhesive plaster
Some individual plasters
Smelling salts
An antiseptic (diluted ready for use)
Petroleum jelly
Tweezers
Aerosol pain killing spray
Crushed ice or cold packs
Disposable gloves
Towel

I.C.E.R.

I.C.E.R. puts in a short form the principles of initial treatment, namely, ice, compression and elevation followed by rest, and these are normally the only methods applied for the first 48 hours after an injury. These should be applied as soon as possible after the injury has taken place because this restricts the development of inflammation and consequently limits oedema in the area.

Ice—packs should not be applied directly to the skin of the area but on top of wet towels or petroleum jelly or oil. This prevents ice burns. Crushed ice is the ideal material but when this is not available gel bags, having been suitably treated in the refrigerator, or frozen peas, offer reasonable alternatives. When it is necessary to transport these they should be carried in a thermal bag. If none of the above are available, then towels wrung out in water as cold as is available provide another solution.

Many people feel that the old method of alternating hot and cold water is very effective. This is achieved by having a pail of water as hot as can be reasonably borne and another pail of water as cold as possible. The area involved is immersed in the cold water for two minutes, taken out and plunged into the hot water for one minute and then back into the cold, repeating for some ten or more minutes. If the area involved is not suitable to be immersed, a similar effect can be achieved by hot and cold towels. When it is necessary and possible the cold treatment may be continued for five minutes in every hour up to a total of 48 hours.

Compression—this is normally achieved by firm bandaging or by applying elastic plaster. The aim is to contain the swelling and this requires a certain amount of expertise because the bandaging must not be so tight as to be restrictive of the circulation but it must be firm enough to achieve its object. The method sometimes used is to bandage the area and then to pour cold water over it. This causes the bandage to shrink slightly and therefore tighten up. The advantage of this method is that when the heat of the body has evaporated the water and the bandage beings to stretch again, more water may be poured on, and so on. Readers should practice the art of bandaging and learn spica bandaging, if the opportunity exists. This form of bandaging provides the necessary compression and support without unduly restricting movement.

Elevation—where possible an injured limb should be elevated so that the blood flows more readily towards the heart. This reduces the pressure caused by fluids in the injured area.

It is generally agreed that cold, compression and elevation are the only desirable treatments for the first 48 hours and during this time the muscle injuries in particular should not be heated, massaged, stretched or electro-stimulated.

Heat treatments

Heat is normally the second stage of the treatment of sports injuries. Heat increases the circulatory flow by dilating the blood vessels and acts as an analgesic by relaxing the muscles.

Infra-red or radiant heat—for technical information see Chapter 16.

Treatment times are not critical but are normally between twenty and thirty minutes. The heat is directed straight on to the skin—that is, all bandages and plasters must be removed and the skin must be free of oil, creams and embrocation. The lamp should be placed at a distance from the skin where it is comfortably warm but not hot, particular care being taken with diabetic patients who have lessened sensitivity to heat and cold. When treating the face, goggles are not necessary but care should be taken, particularly when the heat is applied near the eye, by removing contact lenses and putting pads of cotton wool over the eyes themselves. This form of treatment may be applied several times a day if necessary.

Paraffin wax—the second choice of heat treatment will probably be paraffin wax. It is the second choice only because it requires a little more preparation than infra-red. It has been used in hospitals for many years because the exterior body can tolerate more heat in this form than in practically any other way. Details of preparation and application are to be found in Chapter 13.

Massage

The mechanical effects of massage include the stretching and mobilising of soft tissues, dispersing all the fluids in the area and stimulating the circulatory system. In addition there is the soothing effect of warm hands over the injured area. All remedial massage must be firm, the pressures being such as to achieve the above objectives but without causing any further damage. Normally remedial or Swedish massage is applied with the use of talc as this allows firm contact without sliding, although sometimes when the area is very painful or swollen a suitable oil may be used.

It should also be mentioned that massage before involvement in athletic activity can be very useful and it is here that mechanical massagers of the gyratory type can be of particular value. These have a depth effect which is difficult to achieve by hand, together with a speed that cuts down the time considerably, enabling the therapist to treat a much larger number of people.

If massage is given therapeutically it should be accompanied by suitable exercises. These are normally divided into three stages—passive, active and resistive. Passive is when the movement is applied by the therapist without any help from the patient. Active is when both patient and therapist work together to produce the movement. Resistive is when the patient tries to prevent the movement applied by the therapist—this stage comes, of course, in the final part of the treatment.

Faradism

For technical information on faradism the reader is referred to Chapter 15.

Faradism is useful because it stimulates the muscles without producing any chemical changes. Faradic current is very similar to the form of energy which flows down a motor nerve and is used for the same effect, that is to operate the muscle. It is, therefore, a passive form of exercise, the speed and power both being regulated by the therapist. In this way it is possible to increase the tonus of a muscle to speed up its rehabilitation.

Most modern instruments are equipped with variable surge speed and controllable power. The surge speed indicates the number of times the muscle is activated and this can vary between, say, 5 times a minute and 100 times a minute. Very weak or debilitated muscles are normally worked at the very slow speeds and the rate increased as the muscle improves to a normal maximum of 50 to 60 movements per minute.

Generally, faradism is used once a day. In special circumstances it can be applied two or three times. Faradism may also be used for muscle prognosis, thus determining whether the muscle is improving or retrograding under treatment. For this purpose special electrodes are used, not the normal pads which are usually supplied with faradic instruments, and the amount of current required to move the muscle is measured. If more current than previously is needed to move the muscle, it is retrogressing, whilst if less current is used then it is improving. Such a measurement, of course, requires accurate knowledge of the origin and insertion of the muscle concerned.

There are many multi-output instruments on the market but these are rarely necessary for the sports therapist; a small instrument having two to four outputs is all that is required. If the instrument is only to be used in a static situation then the choice will obviously be a mains instrument, the battery-operated type being the choice of the visiting practitioner.

It should be pointed out that normally faradic treatment may only be applied after consultation with the patient's doctor.

VACUUM SUCTION

This is dealt with in detail in Chapter 14.

Although many people associate vacuum suction with slimming techniques, it should be pointed out that its use for this purpose is of reasonably recent origin, suction cups having been used for thousands of years for their therapeutic value.

The therapeutic effects of vacuum suction include an increased blood and lymph flow, stimulated metabolism and the production of a satisfactory hyperaemia. It has been used successfully for muscle toning, post-traumatic circulatory disorders and has proved particularly valuable in the reduction of oedema. As a treatment form it can prove invaluable for such conditions as bursitis, synovitis, epicondylitis and all those inflammatory conditions which are accompanied by oedema. In working over painful areas a very low vacuum should be used, say 5 per cent, gradually increasing to a maximum of not more than 15 per cent when pain has completely disappeared. Treatment is accelerated when the area has been previously heated, for example, with a radiant heat lamp. To be effective, treatment should be applied once a day.

General conclusions

It is necessary to bring together a number of interrelated points which may be of value to the sports therapist.

When dealing with serious injuries it is important to get the patient to hospital as quickly as possible. Whilst giving immediate aid do not neglect to depute someone to telephone for the ambulance. It is also a general rule relating to serious injuries that the patient should be moved as little as possible—this particularly applies to suspected fractures of the spine, where the patient should not be moved at all before the arrival of medical help. This rule must be observed even if it requires stopping the game or activity in progress.

Fitness—mention has already been made of the importance of prevention of injuries and here fitness plays a very essential role. It must be remembered that the quality of exercise is more important than its quantity. A little regular exercise is more valuable than a large amount taken spasmodically. Two miles jogging or cycling a day, every day, is much better than ten miles on Sunday.

Age factors must also be taken into account. The more vigorous forms of sport, like squash, may be appropriate to younger persons, but exercises such as swimming and walking will certainly be more suitable for older people. Middle-aged people should not undertake jogging before receiving a check-up from their doctor, after which properly cushioned footwear is essential. If possible, the jogging should be done on grass or soft surfaces rather than on concrete. It is advisable to eliminate the competitive spirit, that is not to put a time limit on the covering of a particular circuit and not to be obsessive. In other words, the body should be listened to, especially when it indicates that abstinence from this form of activity is advisable.

Another valuable form of exercise is provided by exercising bicycles and rowing exercisers. With these it is possible to provide suitable programmes for all ages.

Sterlising procedures—it is appreciated that such procedures are very difficult on the sports field but on returning to the centre all items which have been used should be suitably treated. Scissors and tweezers should be immersed in surgical spirit or a strong solution of Dettol. Disposable items should preferably be burned and other items such as gel bags should be thoroughly cleaned with antiseptic solution. Any items which have been used out of the therapist's sports kit should be replaced so that it is ready for immediate use.

Chapter 21

Ultrasound and its use in treatment

PRODUCTION OF ULTRASOUND WAVES

The first thing to make clear is that ultrasonic waves are not part of the electromagnetic spectrum in the way that short waves or microwaves are. Although they are electrically produced, ultrasonic waves are compression waves. The phenomenon of an aircraft breaking through the sound barrier is well known to most people, though not everyone understands exactly what happens. An aircraft in flight produces a lot of noise and this noise travels ahead of it at speeds that vary with the height of the aircraft. Assume that the aircraft is travelling at a height at which the sound waves that it produces travel at 650 miles per hour—if the aircraft itself is travelling at 500 miles per hour, the waves will be travelling 150 miles per hour faster than the aircraft so there is no possibility of the aircraft overtaking them. However, when the aircraft exceeds 650 miles per hour it will catch up with and pass through the sound waves which it has itself produced. These compressed waves form an almost solid wall which the aircraft pushes aside as it passes through, causing the first crack noise that we hear. After the aircraft has passed through the waves they join together again causing the second crack noise. Designers of supersonic planes are therefore very concerned not only with ensuring that the strength of the aircraft is sufficient to allow it to pass through the sound waves, but also that the aircraft will produce as little resistance as possible in breaking the sound waves apart.

If a rod of ferro-electric metal is magnetised by means of an electric current, one end becomes the north pole and the other becomes the south pole. The north and south poles attract each other, so the rod will become fractionally shorter when the current passes. If the applied current is switched rapidly on and off, greater alteration in the length of the rod is produced. In other words the rod will be vibrating, and the vibrations will produce waves of sound. When the same principle is applied to a suitably cut quartz crystal, it will vibrate at very high speeds and so produce ultrasound.

In contrast to electromagnetic radiation, for example, ultrasound is not able to travel in a vacuum. Its speed through different materials varies considerably as will be shown by the following approximate travel speeds:

air	300 m/s
fresh water	1400 m/s
sea water	1500 m/s
muscular tissue	1400 m/s
fatty tissue	1600 m/s

In the early machines the current applied to the crystal face was generated by means of valves and this, combined with the type of mounting used for the crystal in the very large heads used at that time, involved the production of a good deal of heat which meant that the head had to be watercooled. The early instruments were very large (about the size of a small desk) and could only be operated on a site where running water was readily available. Most of these problems have now been overcome—modern instruments are transistorised and the heads are very much smaller so that cooling is no longer necessary and the instruments themselves are very compact and portable.

ULTRA SOUND
TREATMENT UNIT

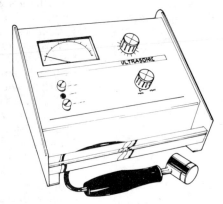

Some confusion is created by instruments advertised as 'audio-sonic', i.e. sound producing. These small units are percussors and not in any way related to the instruments described in this chapter.

EFFECTS

It is generally agreed that ultrasound energy applied to the human body has four types of effect:

(1) Mechanical
(2) Chemical or biological
(3) Thermal
(4) Neural.

Mechanical effects

The main mechanical effect is really micro-massage. Massage as a form of physical medicine has been used for very many centuries—certainly since the days of Hippocrates and probably earlier. Massage in general terms exerts a series of pressures on body tissue and then release them, thus relaxing the tissue.

As has already been seen, ultrasound also produces pressures and when these are applied to the human body they compress and release the tissue as in massage but at very much faster speeds. Also, because of the speed, they are able to effect a micro-massage on tissue which would not produce a response to hand massage. Additionally, because of the controllability of the energy, it is possible to apply ultrasonic massage to areas which would be too painful to hand massage.

Another effect of these very fast sound waves is the oscillation of particles within the energy field. This is generally believed to improve the blood circulation and lymphatic drainage of the site treated, as well as loosening or disintegrating granules associated with rheumatic conditions.

Chemical or Biological Effects

There are a number of chemical effects created by ultrasound waves and it is not the purpose of this chapter to go into these in detail. It will therefore be sufficient to list the more measurable biological reactions so that readers who are interested in such physiological effects will be acquainted with the primary processes involved. It has been noted that the following chemical effects can be attributed to ultrasound irradiation:

(1) Improved permeability of all membranes to sodium and potassium ions.
(2) Inhibition of inflammatory processes.
(3) Vaso dilation.
(4) Analgesia.
(5) A change of tissue pH.
(6) Liberation of homochronologically active materials—transport of ions (see the section on phonophoresis later in this chapter).
(7) Improved hyperaemia.

Thermal Effects

The thermal or heat effect of ultrasound waves is really a by-product, but none the less a very important one. The heat is produced by the friction created by the waves passing through the tissue. The advantage of this form of thermal activity against others in common use is that it is target heat. Infra-red, short wave and microwave have a more general heating effect on the whole of an area whereas ultrasound may be directed at the lesion itself.

Neural Effects

It is a well known fact that the nervous system responds readily to external stimuli as shown by the effects of galvanism, faradism etc. The treatment of the nervous system, and in particular the treatment of

autonomic processes, with ultrasound waves is in its
infancy and—again—it is not the purpose of this
chapter to explain how neural effects are achieved,
but it would appear that ultrasound waves are
stimulating or exciting to the processes involved. As
readers will already know, the autonomic system has
two branches—the sympathetic and the parasympathetic—and irradiation of the corresponding
segments and spinal nerve roots produce somewhat
different results. For example, stimulation of the
sympathetic system raises blood pressure and blood
sugar level, causes sweating and excites secretion of
adrenalin, whereas stimulation of the parasympathetic system retards the heart, promotes
secretion of insulin and lowers blood sugar level.

In arriving at a conclusion as to how the excitation
actually takes place it is well worth considering a
hypothesis based on the discoveries of Professor
Eiichifukada of Tokyo University. He reports that
large molecules such as protein or cellulose exhibit
the piezoelectric effect when subjected to pressure.
This produces electric charges on their surfaces and it
could be that sound pressure produced by ultrasound
waves causes the large molecules to develop a
piezoelectric charge which, in turn, stimulates nerves
as well as muscles.

Although the four types of effect of ultrasound
irradiation are described separately above, this is not
intended to suggest that they are independent in
action. Experience shows that a combination of each
of the four effects is involved in most of the cures or
improvements attributed to ultrasound treatment.

METHODS OF APPLICATION

Early ultrasound instruments were equipped with
very large heads delivering, in many cases, a great
deal of power. This resulted not only in unnecessary
heat but sometimes in unpleasant side-effects because
of the destructive nature of the high energy used.
However, much research and experience has shown
that a safe maximum wattage is 3 W/cm^2 delivered to
a head of 5 cm^2. This gives a total usable energy of
15 W though, as will be seen later, this maximum is
rarely used. However, this is considered to be a safe
maximum, subject of course, as in all physical
treatments, to such warning signals as pain.

As has already been seen, ultrasound waves are
largely ineffective in air as they travel slowly through
this medium but they do travel well through water
and body tissue. It is highly important, therefore, that
there should be no air space between the treatment
head and the body. For this purpose, the site to be
treated is covered with a suitable coupling material to
enable the head not only to move easily but to

eliminate air. Sometimes liquid paraffin or a massage oil is used as a coupling material. This has, of course, good viscosity and allows the head to travel easily but because of its lack of bulk it does not fill up all the cracks and spaces on the surface of the body and is, therefore, not an ideal coupling material. Most manufacturers sell a cream or gel which is comparatively inexpensive and has been especially designed for the coupling purpose.

SOUND HEAD WITHOUT
COUPLING MATERIAL—
AIR SPACE PRESENT

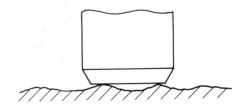

SOUND HEAD WITH
COUPLING MATERIAL—
AIR SPACE ELIMINATED

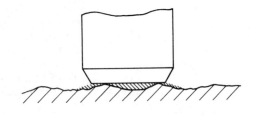

A very satisfactory method of treating uneven surfaces such as feet and hands is the water bath method. Here the extremity is placed in a bath of water, a Schnee bath or similar, and the treatment head is also placed in the water and directed at the lesion site. The distance between the head and the skin can be up to 10 cm although it is more usual to keep the head about 2 cm away from the treatment area. Care should be taken to avoid direct contact between the head and the skin under water. When warm tap water is used in the bath, air bubbles will separate out after a short while and adhere to the skin and the treatment head. As ultrasound does not travel well through air, these bubbles will impede treatment and they should be removed. If purified or well-boiled water is used this procedure becomes unnecessary.

WATER BATH

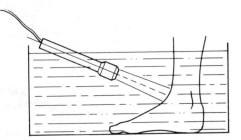

Whilst the water bath method is suitable for the extremities, the irregular shape of the spine also requires special consideration. It is not normally possible to immerse the whole of the spine in water when giving treatment, so a coupling cushion is involved. The coupling cushion is made of plastic film or thin rubber and filled with degassed water to at least 80–90 per cent of the bag's capacity, enabling it to be moulded to the part to be treated. The part is then covered with the normal coupling cream and the coupling cushion is put in position and held there by two fingers of the therapist's hand. The upper surface of the cushion is then covered with cream and the head of the ultrasonic unit is applied to this and used in the ordinary way.

Most instruments are now supplied with two modes of operation—continuous mode and pulsed mode. As the name implies, continuous mode means that the current is continuous and uninterrupted whereas with pulsed mode the energy is pulsed in periods stated by the manufacturers, such as one on – one off, or one on – four off. In the latter, for every 10 ms of the operation the energy would be on for 2 ms and off for 8 ms. Pulsed energy is particularly valuable for treating recent injuries where periostal pain might become intolerable if the current was applied continuously. Many therapists, however, prefer to use continuous current on old, established lesions because they argue that the normal method of contact treatment, which is to move the head in small circles, has the effect of interrupting the energy over any particular point. The pulsed mode should, however, be used in all those cases where it is important that there should be no build up of heat, because the rest period between the bursts of output enables the circulation to cool the area.

CHOICE OF FREQUENCY

We now come to the choice of frequency and here it is important to remember that the higher the frequency, the smaller the depth of penetration. So, conversely—the lower the frequency, within certain limits, the higher the depth of penetration. It should be emphasised that there is no apparent difference in the effect of the treatment when given with, say, 1 MHz or 3 MHz. The only difference is to be found in the depth of penetration. An ultrasonic beam does not terminate, it goes on with ever decreasing power in much the same way as a light beam does. In ultrasound treatment the energy is considered to have lost most of its effectiveness when the tissue through which it is passed reduces its power to half. Without going into the complicated physics involved in these measurements, it is approximately correct to say that for the same power or energy output, 3 MHz only effectively penetrates about one third of the distance that 1 MHz does. With the same power, 1 MHz would penetrate to a depth of 5 cm compared with about 1.4 cm penetration with 3 MHz. Because of this, most manufacturers have now concentrated on the production of instruments which operate at or around 1 MHz. A few manufacturers provide the alternative frequency of 3 MHz, particularly for the benefit of people who specialise in treatment of the skin or the immediate subcutaneous tissue, where depth effect is not so important.

As has already been indicated most instruments now are designed to deliver a maximum of 3 W/cm^2 and they are all fitted with control knobs which give a selection of power outputs varying from as low as 0.1 W/cm^2 to the maximum of 3 W/cm^2. Practitioners will quickly find the power output which is the most suitable for their specialities. It is normally considered wise to operate at somewhere between 1 and 1.5 W/cm^2.

TREATMENT INDICATIONS

It is not the purpose of this chapter, nor is it possible, to provide a complete list of all the conditions which can be treated by ultrasound. The Erlangen Ultrasonic Conference in 1949 reviewed over 100 000 treatments and since then much water has flowed under the bridge. Many more cases and types of case will be on file as having received beneficial effects from insonation. Some guidelines, however, are obviously of value and the following list of conditions with their treatment times and the amount of energy used, should give practitioners a reasonably accurate idea of the range of conditions for which this form of treatment is suitable.

It is now generally accepted that in all cases of trauma where physical medicine would normally be indicated, ultrasonic therapy may be applied immediately after the trauma has occurred. This stimulates the absorption of oedema and starts a cycle around the injured structures which reduces pain, decreases muscle spasm and this, in turn, further reduces the pain level. Normal movements can be performed almost at once, resulting in minimal residual waste products and ensuring that a very low level of fibrous tissue is laid down. This applies especially to severe sprains and strains of muscle fibres, tendons and ligaments, dislocations and fractures, acute tenosynovitis, tendinitis, synovitis and capsulitis. In all these conditions pulsed ultrasound is indicated because of the possible high pain level.

Examples
of treatment

Condition	Traumatic synovitis
Intensity	0.75–1.00 W
Mode	Pulse
Duration	3 min
Note	Twice daily
Condition	Ligament injuries
Intensity	1.00–1.25 W
Mode	Continuous
Duration	Up to 5 min
Note	Every other day
Condition	Contusions
Intensity	1.00–1.25 W
Mode	Continuous
Duration	5 min
Note	Twice on day of injury—once a day thereafter
Condition	Sprains, strains
Intensity	1.00 W
Mode	Pulse or continuous
Duration	5 min
Note	Twice daily; choose pulse or continuous according to pain level
Condition	Metasalgia
Intensity	1.00–1.25 W
Mode	Continuous
Duration	5 min
Note	In water bath
Condition	Torn muscles or ligaments
Intensity	1.00 W
Mode	Pulse or continuous
Duration	5 min
Note	Twice on day of injury—once a day thereafter
Condition	Fractures where the splints are removable
Intensity	1.00 W
Mode	Pulse
Duration	5 min
Note	Daily
Condition	Frozen shoulder
Intensity	1.00–1.50 W
Mode	Continuous or pulse
Duration	3 min
Note	Every other day
Condition	Fibrositis
Intensity	1.00–1.50 W
Mode	Continuous
Duration	5 min
Note	Every other day

Condition	Rheumatoid arthritis
Intensity	1.00 W
Mode	Continuous
Duration	3 min
Note	Twice a week

Condition	Brachial neuritis
Intensity	0.75–1.00 W
Mode	Continuous
Duration	5 min
Note	Daily

Condition	Sciatic neuritis
Intensity	1.00 W
Mode	Pulse
Duration	2 min
Note	Daily

Condition	Bronchial asthma
Intensity	1.00–1.50 W
Mode	Continous
Duration	2 min
Note	Along subclavian stellate ganglion

Condition	Keloids
Intensity	1.50 W
Mode	Continuous
Duration	5 min
Note	Twice a week

Condition	Herpes zosta
Intensity	1.00 W
Mode	Continuous or pulse
Duration	3 min
Note	Every other day

Condition	Bursitis
Intensity	1.00 W
Mode	Pulse or continuous
Duration	3 min
Note	Daily

CONTRA-INDICATIONS

For the instrument

The energy should not be switched on until you are ready to use the instrument, that is when the treatment head is either in contact with the patient or in a water bath. Allowing the treatment head to operate in free air for any length of time is likely to result in damage.

For the patient

The following contra-indications are given purely as a guide. Many authorities differ considerably on what they consider to be dangerous uses of ultrasound. For example, while the majority would not use sound waves over the heart, there are some who use them specifically to treat heart conditions. As the maxim 'if in doubt—don't' is particularly applicable to physical medicine, the following list of contra-indications may be considered unless or until experience and increased knowledge invalidates them.

  Over the cardiac region
  In cardio-vascular conditions such as thrombosis and phlebitis
  Over the brain
  Over the eyes
  Over the reproductive organs
  Over the abdomen, especially in the case of pregnant women because of the risk of abortion
  Over tumours, whether benign or malignant
  In cases of acute sepsis
  In cases of acute inflammation, e.g. osteomyelitis
  Over carbuncles or boils
  In cases of pulmonary or bone tuberculosis
  On patients suffering from haemophilia or hyperthyroidism

No patient should continue to receive ultrasound treatment at the same energy level after complaining of excess heat, a burning sensation or pain. This indicates that the upper limits of tolerance have been reached and the treatment should be immediately modified—that is, the energy should be reduced to a point where these reactions do not re-occur.

PHONOPHORESIS

Phonophoresis is one of the very valuable treatments available with ultrasound, but its use developed slowly. Although early work was done in this field by the Germans it was—to an extent—neglected in favour of the more usual physiotherapy type of treatment.

Reference has already been made in this book (p. 140) to iontophoresis or ionisation by means of a galvanic current. This causes charged particles to move along a path from one electrode to the other, but electrically neutral particles are not affected. The limitation of this form of treatment is that only certain substances (those carrying positive or negative charges) can effectively be introduced into the system.

Ultrasound does not suffer from these dis-advantages because, being non-electrical, it does not dissociate the molecule in any way. By its sheer unidirectional power it is able to force the whole molecule into the tissue, and this process is known as phonophoresis. There is no way in which it is possible to introduce the whole molecule into the system using electrophoresis.

In addition to its medical uses, beauty therapists have found this method of considerable value when they wish to introduce beauty preparations into subcutaneous tissue. As a general guide, for sub-cutaneous treatments an intensity of 0.75–1.00 W and a treatment time of about five minutes should be sufficient. For joints and deep-seated penetration a higher intensity will be needed and this should be pulsed in order to prevent a heat build-up in the tissue which could, in certain circumstances, interfere with the treatment.

OTHER USES OF ULTRASOUND

Some of the other uses of ultrasound are commercial, others are of defence value or of use in science and perhaps especially in medicine—that is, general medicine or surgery as opposed to physical medicine which has been dealt with in the previous chapters.

The speed of the agitations made possible by ultrasound equipment means that it is used extensively by pharmaceutical and chemical companies for mixing paints and other materials. Sonar equipment, as used by the navy for detecting underwater objects such as submarines, is very well known. It is also used for detecting faults in the metal plates of ships and metal fatigue in aircraft. Ultrasound has also been used to clean clothes, the dirt particles being vibrated out of the fibres, thus avoiding the need for the chemicals used in normal dry cleaning.

The other particular value which ultrasound has in medicine is in sonography. This is the use of ultrasound energy to take 'photographs' of the interior of the body, in much the same way that X-rays are used, but without some of the damaging effects which are associated with X-rays. This is particularly of value in determining the exact position of, for example, a baby in the womb—a diagnosis which medicine has been reluctant in the past to achieve with X-rays because of the possible damage to the baby. The ultrasound method is now widely used in maternity departments and enables doctors, for the first time, to study actual pictures of the baby's beating heart before it is born and also to locate malignancies or deformities. This means that the necessary medical action can be taken. The technique is completely painless and has no harmful effects on either mother or baby.

Part IV

Management of Patient and Practice

The preceding chapters have been devoted to providing the physical therapist with the knowledge which is necessary to undertake treatments. In other words, an understanding of the body and how it works; what may go wrong with it and how physical therapy may accelerate those physiological processes necessary for the body to return to a state of normality and health.

The physical therapist is, however, a professional person and this involves much more than just the knowledge and expertise acquired from basic training. The following section endeavours to fill in some of those gaps and to help the therapist to become a responsible, successful member of an honourable profession.

Chapter 22

Patient Assessment

You will note that this chapter is headed 'Patient Assessment' and that the word 'diagnosis' is not used. Diagnosis is the province of the properly qualified medical person.

The physical therapist's assessment is very important and it is equally important to record that assessment correctly. A good therapist learns how to observe accurately and to note any abnormality. Observation in this sense is not only done by means of the eyes but with the nose, ear and hand. The nose will detect any unusual odour, for example, diabetes is sometimes associated with sweet smelling breath which will enable the therapist to take the necessary precautions in treatment, especially heat treatments. The ear will detect any unusual breathing sound and panting or bronchitic breathing will make the therapist proceed with extreme caution. Also, when massaging the patient the fingers should be taught to automatically flash back to the brain anything unusual in the body structure, a protuberance that does not correspond to a normal anatomical one, or a rise in temperature on a particular part of the skin suggesting inflammation, or increased sensitivity. When such abnormalities are found they must be referred back to the patient's medical adviser before treatment of the part is undertaken.

However, assuming that the patient has already been given a diagnosis or alternatively that they are coming in for general treatment such as toning or relaxation treatment, then it is necessary to record the patient's requirements, and certainly in the case of slimming treatment it is necessary to have certain statistical records. These records must, of necessity, vary according to the type of clinic or practice in which the therapist is involved and the following two examples could be applied, in the first instance to the clinic which primarily exists for slimming support treatments, and in the second, to the clinic which has numerous medical referrals.

Example 1

date, name, address, telephone number, age, sex, reason for coming, therapist's observations and on the other side of the card in vertical columns: date, height, weight, bust, waist, abdomen, hips, thighs and a blank column.

Example 2

date, name, address, telephone number, age, sex, occupation, name of doctor, brief medical history, what drugs have been taken and for how long, therapist's observations.

The information required by the first one could easily be put on an index card whilst the second one requires a larger card or index sheet.

POINTS TO NOTE WHEN MAKING AN ASSESSMENT

The patient should be weighed either in the nude or with a minimum of clothing. The first reason for this is that the weight of the clothing can easily alter from visit to visit—secondly—observing the patient in a state of undress enables the therapist to see more clearly the body structure, posture, large fat folds, etc. Weighing is not normally recommended more than once a week and it should preferably be done at the same time of the day. In the case of the female patient allowance should be made for the monthly cycle because many women put on extra weight (due to water retention) in the immediate premenstrual part of the cycle. Their weight can go up as much as 2–3 kg though the average increase is probably 1 kg.

As a guide to the therapist the following tables help to establish a target weight. These tables are based on those of life assurance companies and show the *maximum* desirable weight relative to height and frame. All the weights given are for the naked body.

The formula for establishing the frame category is as follows:

Take the width of the ribs laterally (in the axilla region) and the width of the hips laterally at the widest point. Add these together, multiply by 2 and add 13 for women or 19 for men. If this total approximately equals the height in inches, this is a *medium* frame. If the total is two or more inches less than the height, then the frame is small. Two or more inches greater and the frame is *large*. A pelvimeter which is normally used for determining pelvic size is an excellent instrument for taking these measurements.

Maximum Weight Desirable for Women

Height		Small		Medium		Large	
4' 11"	1.50 m	7 st. 4 lb	46.3 kg	7 st. 13 lb	50.3 kg	8 st. 11 lb	55.8 kg
5' 0"	1.52 m	7 st. 5 lb	47.7 kg	8 st. 2 lb	51.7 kg	9 st. 0 lb	57.1 kg
5' 1"	1.55 m	7 st. 10 lb	49.0 kg	8 st. 5 lb	53.0 kg	9 st. 3 lb	58.5 kg
5' 2"	1.57 m	7 st. 13 lb	50.3 kg	8 st. 9 lb	54.9 kg	9 st. 7 lb	60.3 kg
5' 3"	1.60 m	8 st. 2 lb	51.7 kg	8 st. 13 lb	56.7 kg	9 st. 11 lb	62.1 kg
5' 4"	1.63 m	8 st. 6 lb	53.4 kg	9 st. 4 lb	59.0 kg	10 st. 1 lb	63.9 kg
5' 5"	1.65 m	8 st. 10 lb	55.3 kg	9 st. 10 lb	61.7 kg	10 st. 5 lb	65.8 kg
5' 6"	1.68 m	9 st. 0 lb	57.1 kg	9 st. 12 lb	62.6 kg	10 st. 9 lb	67.6 kg
5' 7"	1.70 m	9 st. 4 lb	59.0 kg	10 st. 2 lb	64.4 kg	10 st. 13 lb	69.4 kg
5' 8"	1.73 m	9 st. 9 lb	61.2 kg	10 st. 6 lb	66.2 kg	11 st. 4 lb	71.5 kg
5' 9"	1.75 m	9 st. 13 lb	63.0 kg	10 st. 10 lb	67.9 kg	11 st. 9 lb	73.8 kg
5' 10"	1.78 m	10 st. 3 lb	64.9 kg	11 st. 0 lb	69.7 kg	12 st. 1 lb	76.7 kg

Maximum Weight Desirable for Men

Height		Small		Medium		Large	
5′ 3″	1.60 m	8 st. 6 lb	53.4 kg	9 st. 2 lb	58.0 kg	10 st. 0 lb	63.5 kg
5′ 4″	1.63 m	8 st. 9 lb	54.9 kg	9 st. 5 lb	59.4 kg	10 st. 4 lb	65.3 kg
5′ 5″	1.65 m	8 st. 13 lb	56.7 kg	9 st. 9 lb	61.2 kg	10 st. 8 lb	67.2 kg
5′ 6″	1.68 m	9 st. 3 lb	58.5 kg	9 st. 13 lb	63.0 kg	10 st. 13 lb	69.4 kg
5′ 7″	1.70 m	9 st. 7 lb	60.3 kg	10 st. 4 lb	65.3 kg	11 st. 4 lb	71.5 kg
5′ 8″	1.73 m	9 st. 11 lb	62.1 kg	10 st. 8 lb	67.2 kg	11 st. 8 lb	73.3 kg
5′ 9″	1.75 m	10 st. 2 lb	64.4 kg	10 st. 12 lb	69.0 kg	11 st. 12 lb	75.2 kg
5′ 10″	1.78 m	10 st. 6 lb	66.2 kg	11 st. 3 lb	71.1 kg	12 st. 3 lb	77.5 kg
5′ 11″	1.80 m	10 st. 10 lb	67.9 kg	11 st. 8 lb	73.3 kg	12 st. 8 lb	79.9 kg
6′ 0″	1.83 m	11 st. 0 lb	69.7 kg	11 st. 11 lb	74.8 kg	12 st. 13 lb	82.3 kg
6′ 1″	1.85 m	11 st. 5 lb	72.1 kg	12 st. 2 lb	77.1 kg	13 st. 4 lb	86.2 kg
6′ 2″	1.88 m	11 st. 9 lb	73.8 kg	12 st. 7 lb	79.4 kg	13 st. 9 lb	88.4 kg
6′ 3″	1.90 m	11 st. 11 lb	74.8 kg	13 st. 0 lb	82.6 kg	14 st. 0 lb	90.7 kg

Measurements should be taken with the tape just snugly fitting over the part being measured, not tight enough to create an indentation in the fat nor loose enough for the tape to sag. With practice the right amount of tightness can be achieved so avoiding the very common error of false measurements.

In noting the medical history (this is normally limited to those conditions likely to be affected by physical therapy) take particular note of operations, accidents and cardio-vascular troubles. If the patient volunteers the information that he/she is taking drugs or other medications, the therapist should find out which ones, why and for how long.

When patients come specifically for slimming support treatment it is interesting to note whether he/she is currently on a diet, has been on a diet in the past or was never on a diet. It might also be worth noting whether the patient has been overweight since childhood, puberty, marriage, first child or menopause in the case of a female or, in the case of a male, since the age of approximately twenty, thirty, forty or fifty.

Under the heading 'occupation' many are self-explanatory and give a good idea as to whether the patient is likely to be standing for most of the day or sitting for most of the day with a lot or little exercise. When a patient puts an occupation such as 'housewife' it might be worthwhile exploring her other activities to find out whether she plays golf, walks, gardens, rides, etc.

Under the heading 'reason for coming' it is usual to note any special instructions which the doctor may have given.

Finally, either on the case history sheet or, more usually, on a separate card, a record must be kept of the patient's attendances, the dates, the treatment being received on those dates and the amount paid or to be charged.

The above ideas are given purely as guides. They indicate the kind of information required and should enable the therapist to produce a case history sheet or card index particularly appropriate to his/her type of practice or clinic. Whichever form is finally adopted it cannot be over-emphasised that the keeping of adequate records is an integral part of professional life.

Chapter 23

Clinic Organisation and Management

This chapter is aimed at helping newly qualified therapists in the course of setting up a practice or those who are expecting to occupy a position of management in someone else's employ.

It is stressed that rules and regulations vary from country to country, state to state and even county to county. It is therefore important to regard this chapter as a general guide rather than a statement of facts. It should, however, help the therapist to identify the main areas in which advice needs to be obtained from a professional or from the local authority.

PREMISES

Having located premises which appear suitable for the purpose of establishing a clinic, it should be ascertained whether consent has been given for the purpose to which they are to be put. In the United Kingdom this comes under the Department of Town and Country Planning—of which there are offices in most of the large centres of population. In most other countries there are similar bodies.

Following a change in the law in early 1982 it is no longer necessary to register a business name. All that is required (when the name under which the business is trading is not your own personal name) is that the name of the business plus the name and address of the owner must be put on to a card and placed where it may easily be seen by persons visiting the premises.

In addition, most countries require a licence to practise and information about this may be obtained from the Department of Health, Medical Officers of Health, Department of Public Control or Department of the Environment. In the United Kingdom application is normally made to the Chief Trading Standards Officer or the Environmental Health Officer who advise the therapist of their requirements for the area. The usual stipulations include that the therapist should have graduated from a college or training centre recognised by the Department. The licence granted will only be for work within the areas for which the therapist has documentary evidence of proficiency. The principal areas of treatment are massage, heat treatments (including sauna), electrical treatments and ultraviolet ray treatments. The authority will indicate what controls they have on advertising, the publication of prices, requirements for safety, electrical checks and fire precautions and they may, at their discretion, impose limits on the therapies practised. For example the authorities may refuse to include sauna treatments in the licence because of the unsuitability of the building. When a licence has been granted, it is normally renewable yearly and the practice is subject to inspection at any normal time to enable the inspector to ascertain whether it is being run strictly within the terms prescribed by the licence.

Premises on which epilation or ear piercing is carried out have to be registered in the U.K. and are subject to inspection. Some authorities require an annual certificate of safety from a qualified electrician, but in any case it is advisable for regular safety checks to be made on equipment, especially where electricity is concerned.

When the above licence has been obtained but before accepting the first patient—the premises and its contents should be insured including third party indemnity—this is to cover accidents other than those arising out of the treatments, for example, if a person visiting the premises falls down the stairs. Additionally, therapists must have professional public indemnity insurance. This is protection against accidents or injury happening to the patient during the course of treatment and this cover will normally be obtained through the professional body of which the therapist is a member.

The premises are expected to have reasonable toilet and washing facilities for both staff and patients, the provision of a first aid box, fire extinguisher(s) and a free-standing or wall thermometer to indicate that the heating is at a satisfactory level.

EXAMPLE OF LAYOUT OF A CONSULTING ROOM DOUBLING UP FOR TREATMENT

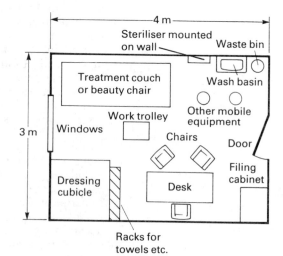

Racks for towels etc.

SETTING UP A PRACTICE

Practices fall generally into two categories: (1) visiting only and (2) clinic. Before embarking on setting up either type it is important to estimate the costs involved. These can be classified under the following headings:

(1) *Capital expenditure*—purchase and preparation of premises (or car), equipment etc.
(2) *Overheads of the premises*—including business rates, rent (if rented or leased property), light, heat, cleaning, laundry etc.
(3) *Expendables*—tissues, paper towels, cosmetics, magazines for waiting room etc.
(4) *Labour*—including an allowance for yourself.
(5) *Publicity*—brochures, price lists, advertising and other public relations.
(6) *Professional services*—e.g. accountant, solicitor.

Capital expenditure is going to be the largest outgoing and for the purposes of preparing an estimate, it should be broken down over a period of five years. All other costs are recurring and should be allowed for.

The possible income generated must be offset against the costs and this is where many new practitioners make mistakes. Although you may be prepared to work eight hours a day, six days a week, fifty weeks a year, it would be foolish to assume that the whole of that time would be filled up with clients. First of all you have to build up a list of clients, but even when this has been achieved you will find many blanks in your appointment book due to clients' holidays, illness (of clients themselves or their dependants) and even bad weather. Established practitioners would be well aware of this situation, but it must not be overlooked by those starting out. The risk is reduced in a visiting practice, but here allowances must be made for travelling time.

If you do not have sufficient personal capital to start a practice, equipment may be purchased on a hire purchase agreement or a loan may be obtained from the bank or building society, but in each of these cases the interest can amount to a large sum and must be allowed for. When borrowing money, especially on hire purchase, it is easy to be influenced by salesmen to buy equipment which is not absolutely essential to the efficient running of the practice. Remember, it is easy to buy additional equipment when current equipment is justifying itself or when new demands arise.

Publicity

You will need a leaflet or brochure setting out your services. This should be concise, including your name, address, telephone number and of course your qualifications. If you are running a clinic, the hours of business should be stated, and if the practice is a visiting one, the area of operation should be given. Reference should be made to any specialities you practice and it is a good idea to give some indication

of costs, at least for your basic treatments.
For example:

Full facial (1 hour)   . . . . .
Body massage (1 hour)   . . . . .
Sports clinic ($\frac{1}{2}$ hour treatment) . . . . .

These brochures should be distributed as widely as possible locally.

Large advertisements in the public press rarely justify the cost, except possibly for special occasions like an opening. However a regular small advertisement in the personal or medical services column of the local weekly paper will keep your name, address and telephone number constantly before the public.

If you are working on your own, an answering machine is a good investment. Your recorded message should be short and to the point and should say that you will phone back as soon as you are free.

National Insurance

Whether you are working for yourself or in a partnership you will have to pay a Class II stamp on a weekly basis. This applies to the United Kingdom, but other countries have comparable systems.

Value Added Tax (VAT)

Each year the Chancellor of the Exchequer sets a minimum annual turnover figure for businesses and when the turnover of a particular business exceeds this figure, all its services and products become VAT rated. This means that VAT (at a set percentage rate) is added to their cost. Since the 1990 budget liability is calculated in retrospect, i.e. on the turnover of the previous year. If a business is registered for VAT, the amount of VAT paid on goods or services bought from other companies can be claimed back from the government.

PAYE

Pay-as-you-earn in the United Kingdom is a statutory system by which the employer is required to deduct the income tax at the time the wages or salary are paid. Each employee will have a P45 form from the previous employer and this form will show the employee's code number, the total remuneration to date and the amount of tax deducted. When the employee leaves your service he/she must be given an updated P45.

Accounts

For tax purposes it is obligatory to keep accounts and in most countries tax laws are so complex it is advisable to employ an accountant, at least for the preparation of the yearly statement for submission to the Inspector of Taxes. The accountant will usually indicate the kind of records he wishes to be kept but, in the absence of such instructions or if the practice commences before an accountant is appointed, it is essential to keep a record of all monies received and paid out. In the case of the outgoings, they should be supported as far as possible by receipted bills or statements with a clear indication of the purpose for which the money was spent. Many expenses are subject to tax relief; in addition to the more obvious ones of rent, light, heat and telephone there are such recurring charges as laundry, cleaning, petrol and car expenses if the practice is a visiting one, provision of magazines for a waiting room and so on. If in doubt as to whether an item is eligible for tax relief or not, include it in your list and leave it to the professional accountant to eliminate it in the event of its being an inadmissible expense. The accountant will also advise you on VAT liability and how to operate the PAYE scheme if you have any employees. If you sell products of any kind you are also expected to have a simple form of stock control.

Contract of Employment

The following information is given only as a guide to the regulations applying in the United Kingdom and generally in the countries of the European Common Market. It is not intended to be comprehensive and if in any doubt please seek professional assistance. Other countries will have their own laws and information about these should be available locally.

If you employ staff you are required to give each employee a written statement of particulars of the terms of employment and this must be done within thirteen weeks of the commencement of work. Such a statement must include the following:

The names of employer and employee
Date when employment began
Scale of remuneration (or method of calculating it)
Whether payment is weekly or monthly
Terms and conditions relating to hours of work
Holiday arrangements
Procedures relating to sickness and injury
Length of notice required by either side
Job title

Dismissal

An employee who has been employed for more than one month but less than two years is entitled to one week's notice. If employed continuously for more than two but less than twelve years, the entitlement is one week for each continuous year of service. For an employee with over twelve years' service not less than twelve weeks notice is required. **Unfair dismissal** is a complex subject which requires legal assistance.

Maternity Leave

This is applicable to employees who have been in continuous employment for at least two years by the eleventh week before confinement.

EQUIPMENT

Specialised forms of equipment have been dealt with in the second part of this book but there is certain basic equipment which is common to most clinics and the following information is given in the hope that it will help the therapist to choose that which is most appropriate to the type of practice envisaged.

Couches

Couches come in a variety of forms. First there is the lightweight or examination couch. This normally has a tilt head and is suitable for most treatments other than massage or manipulation. This is because the legs are bolted on to the frame and not cross supported. Massage couches usually have legs fitted as an integral part of the couch and have cross struts to strengthen them. They cost rather more but they are very much more substantial. Their height is usually 66 cm (26 inches) against the 76 cm (30 inches) of an examination couch. These are also fitted with tilt heads.

MASSAGE COUCH
WITH TILT HEAD

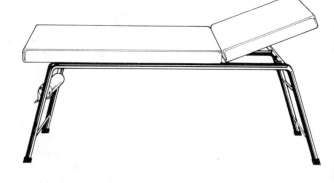

For therapists with visiting practices there is a folding massage couch. This is very strong, is available with a tilt head and when folded will fit into the boot of most small cars.

For the more sophisticated clinic there is the hydraulic couch. This is a very heavily built couch fitted with hydraulic lift, having a maximum height of about 90 cm (36 inches) and a minimum of 50 cm (19 inches). It is constructed from heavy gauge metal, the top being covered with expanded vinyl. The head has a multi-positional tilt.

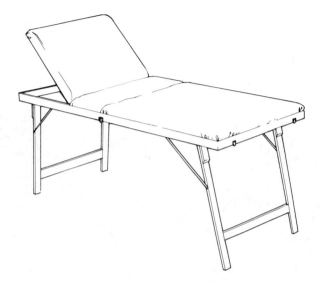

FOLDING MASSAGE
COUCH

The ultimate in couches is the electric lift with a tilt head and, if required, a tilt foot and a cut-out section for the patient's nose when in a prone position. The couch can be supplied with a drop down undercarriage which enables it to be moved about.

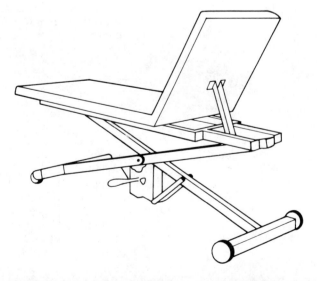

HYDRAULIC COUCH

ELECTRIC LIFT
COUCH

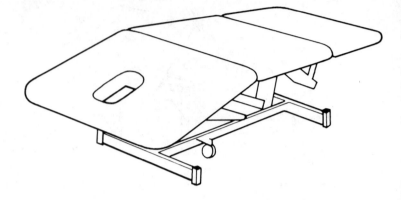

ELECTRIC
MANIPULATION
COUCH

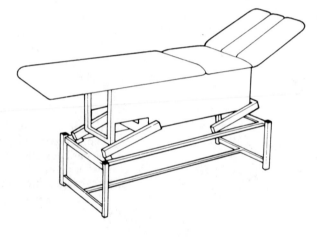

For the therapist requiring a combination unit there is the 'Chouch'. This is mounted on a tubular metal base and is so designed that it can be used as a treatment chair with an adjustable back and leg rest or, with the removal of the arms, as a level massage couch.

'CHOUCH'
(combined treatment
couch and chair)

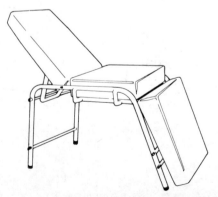

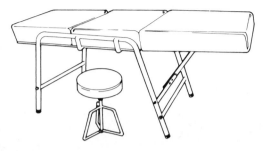

'CHOUCH' IN
MASSAGE POSITION

Treatment Trolleys

These are available in a variety of models; the
simplest one has two glass shelves. They are also
available with guard rails to prevent instruments
from sliding off the back and sides, and with drawers
and cupboards. Usual sizes are 46 × 46 cm
(18 inches × 18 inches), 61 × 46 cm (24 inches × 18
inches) and 76 × 46 × 86 cm (30 inches × 18 inches
× 34 inches) high.

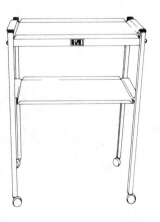

TREATMENT TROLLEY

Scales

Most therapists will be satisfied with low level, large
dial scales; these are comparatively inexpensive in
comparison with the more accurate sliding cursor
scales which are available, if required, with height
measures.

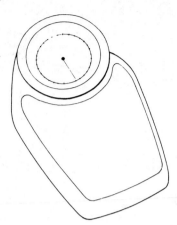

SCALES
(raised dial model)

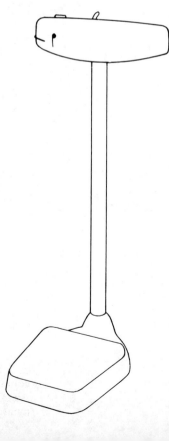

SCALES
(clinical model)

Sterilisers

Cabinet sterilisers suitable for a physical therapy clinic come in two forms and several sizes. The *vapour* type which is the cheaper, and the *ultraviolet ray* type. The latter is suitable for keeping in a sterile condition instruments which have already been cleansed.

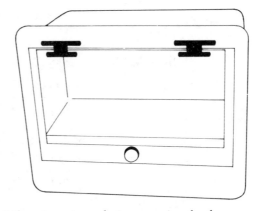

CABINET STERILISER

Where invasive techniques are involved, e.g. electrolysis, particular care has to be taken to avoid infection especially hepatitis and the AIDS virus known as human immunodeficiency virus or HIV. Here ordinary sterilising methods are not sufficient. It is therefore recommended that disposable needles be used. Otherwise needles should be autoclaved or put into a glass-bead type steriliser for a minimum of 20 minutes.

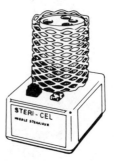

BEAD STERILISER

AIDS

Outside of the body the AIDS virus HIV is easily destroyed by normal disinfectants. The danger occurs when it enters the body via cuts, broken skin or body fluids. If an AIDS victim or HIV-positive person is being treated, in addition to the usual hygiene techniques it is suggested that disposable gloves be worn and disposable towels used. On the termination of the treatment those should be put into a sealed plastic bag. In addition all contact surfaces should be thoroughly sterilised.

Towels

Towels are required for the couch and for patient use and there should be an adequate supply, allowing for laundry time. Paper towels to go on the couch are also available and these will save laundry bills as well as giving an ultra-hygienic appearance.

Gowns

Gowns are generally made from absorbent towelling material which may be purchased in the same colour as the towels.

SUMMARY

Do not enter into any binding agreement regarding property until you have first ascertained that Town and Country Planning consent has been given.

Do not agree to purchase property until it has been professionally surveyed and do not enter into partnership or similar arrangements before taking legal advice.

Professional help may appear expensive at the beginning of a career but it can save a lot of money and headaches later on.

Chapter 24

Professionalism, Ethics and Patient Support

PROFESSIONALISM

It is true to say that the therapist is, in fact, two persons—he is a private *and* a professional person, and the two are indivisible. A doctor is not only a doctor when he is working in a hospital or his surgery but is equally a representative of his profession when he is taking part in sport or leisure activities.

Professionalism is something that is acquired during the long period of training and it is a quality which becomes more marked when graduates have the responsibility of their own patients. There is no quick way of learning professionalism but there are some guidelines to help:

(1) When with the patient give that patient your undivided attention.
(2) Cultivate the art of putting out of your mind your own personal interests or problems.
(3) Forget about the previous patient and just concentrate on the present one.
(4) When the next patient is presented make sure that you do not carry over problems from previous sessions.
(5) Always wear a white coat or other professional uniform and if you are a member of a professional body wear your membership badge. The uniform does more than protect your own clothes—it projects a professional image.
(6) Whether visiting or in your own clinic, always make a point of washing your hands before undertaking treatment and, if possible, do this in such a way that the patient is aware that you have done so.
(7) Never let a patient dictate the treatment nor the form it should take because you are the person who has the necessary knowledge to decide this, though it is reasonable to take into account the patient's preferences.
(8) Talk to the patient but do not gossip.
(9) Please guard against any emotional involvement. This applies not only to problems relating to sex but a whole range of problems which may harass a patient. Give good, sound advice, help with the problem in any way you can but do not become emotionally involved in it.

ETHICS

The following extracts culled from the published code of ethics of two professional bodies indicate very clearly the standard of behaviour which is required from their professionally qualified members.

'Members shall, at all times, conduct their professional lives with the propriety and dignity becoming to a servant of the public and pledge that they will, at all times, place service before self. They also pledge that they will, under no circumstances, infringe the code of morality becoming to their profession and to commit no breach of conduct which will bring grief upon themselves, upon society or upon their fellow practitioners'.

'Members shall confine their services to within recognised spheres of their profession and shall not offer nor promise cures for specific conditions.'

'No member, who having been employed by a therapist, shall on leaving his employ attempt to persuade his former employer's patients to become his patients'.

'No member or Associate who is not a registered Medical Practitioner shall accept patients for medical diagnosis or for the treatment of a medical condition except on reference by a registered Medical Practitioner'.

'All members incur an obligation to uphold the dignity of the profession and they shall at all times act honourably towards their clients and fellow practitioners. They shall at all times maintain professional secrecy and shall refrain from criticising the work of a fellow practitioner'.

To these might be added three practices which are generally accepted:

(1) When a patient is referred by a doctor or other professional person the instructions given at the time of referral must be scrupulously carried out and not added to in any way.
(2) A patient should not be accepted for treatment if being treated by anyone else currently for the same or associated condition.
(3) When you accept a patient you are obligated to give the best treatment of which you are capable irrespective of race, creed or social status.

PATIENT SUPPORT

The very quest for knowledge, which improves skill and efficiency, can easily obscure the biggest single ingredient of success—the patient. However luxurious your clinic, however excellent your treatments and however superb the products you use, they are of no avail if you neglect the opportunity to demonstrate them to the patients.

Patients should take precedence over all other considerations although the other factors may be valuable contributory ones.

Patients usually need understanding, frequently sympathy and often they need convincing that the treatment chosen for them is the right one. Very obviously, if the therapist is able to get the co-operation of the patient, the treatment is likely to be more successful. There is no golden pathway to success in establishing the right relationship and confidence because so much depends on the personalities involved. There are however three considerations which it might be helpful to bear in mind:

(1) The treatment should be such as to be and appear reasonable and the patient should benefit from it.
(2) As far as is possible the patient should enjoy the treatment.
(3) The therapist should appear to be personally involved in the patient's progress.

Under the first heading—it may be necessary to explain in simple terms to patients the nature of the conditions for which they are being treated, followed by a brief description of the treatment they are to receive and its possible or expected results. It is acceptable to quote to the patient results which have been achieved in similar circumstances to his—but be careful not to overstate a case or create false optimism in the patient. From the patient's point of view the treatment should appear to be reasonable and an understanding of exactly what is involved should provide him/her with confidence and hopes of success in his/her case.

Under heading (2), this does not necessarily mean that the treatment will be without some discomfort or pain but rather that the environment and attitudes should contribute to the greatest degree of comfort and peace of mind possible in the circumstances. The couch should be prepared before the patient arrives, and all materials likely to be required during the treatment should be ready. There should be a quiet air of efficiency and absence of rush and bustle and, as far as is possible, freedom from the interference of telephones or other interruptions. Therapists should anticipate, as far as possible, the needs of the patient and do anything that will save him/her from embarrassment.

Patients should be instructed clearly as to how much of their clothing it is necessary to remove, and the position of the changing room and toilet clearly indicated. When the patient is ready for treatment he/she should be assisted on to the couch or treatment chair, the therapist making sure that the patient is lying or sitting in a comfortable position. If the patient has a cold, place a supply of tissues alongside the couch. Should the patient wish to talk make a sincere effort to join in the conversation but if the patient wishes to be quiet then respect this. Under no circumstances should the therapist impose his/her own problems on the patient.

Under heading (3)—a regular weighing and measuring of the patient, done personally by the therapist, helps to elicit a reciprocal responsibility from the patient. When the course of treatment is finished make it clear to the patient that you would like him/her to report in one or two weeks' time to be reweighed or remeasured or for such other checks as you may think necessary to enable you to keep an eye on his/her progress. If he/she does not present him/ herself for this check there is no harm in sending a reminder card or letter similar to the ones that are often used by dentists.

An experienced therapist learns by touch, by speech and perhaps most of all by being a good listener, how to establish a good relationship with the patient and in this way accelerate the healing process.

Conclusion

Most of this book has been devoted to the knowledge of 'why' and 'how' on the basis that when the rationale is understood the decision of 'when, where and how much' is very much easier.

It is important to acquire knowledge and achieve still more expertise but it is even more important that these attributes should be directed by the belief in our own ability to contribute to the relief of pain, the reduction of disease and the restoration of health. The poet, Henry Twells, wrote 'Your touch has still its ancient power, no word from you may fruitless fall, hear in this quiet evening hour and in your mercy heal us all'. This is outside race and creed, beyond sectarianism or political convenience, it is personal dedication to a profession or part of a profession which, from time immemorial, has been dedicated to the service of its fellows, that by your treatment you enable people to face up to life with renewed energy, to regain health or rediscover the joy of living. This is the true reward of the physical therapist.

Some Useful Addresses

Examining Bodies

Examining bodies who have separate Therapy examinations or a Therapy content in their general examinations:

City and Guilds of London Institute,
76 Portland Place, London, W1N 4AA, England.

Confederation of Beauty Therapy and Cosmetology,
2nd Floor, 34 Imperial Square, Cheltenham, Glos.
GL50 1QZ

ITEC—International Therapy Examination Council,
James House, Oakelbrook Mill, Newent, Glos.
GL18 1HD

International Health and Beauty Council,
109 Felpham Road, Felpham, West Sussex PO22 7PW

Professional Organisations

Professional organisations offering their members services which include public indemnity insurance:

British Association of Beauty Therapy and Cosmetology,
2nd Floor, 34 Imperial Square, Cheltenham, Glos.
GL50 1QZ

Independent Professional Therapists' International,
97 London Road, Retford, Notts. DN22 7EB
Tel: 0777 700383

Equipment Suppliers

R.A. Andrew Dodd (Electro-Medical) Ltd.
12 Richmond Place, Brighton, BN2 2NA

Ellisons Ltd.
Crondal Road, Exhall, Coventry, CV7 9NH
Tel: 0203 361619

Taylor Reeson Laboratories Ltd.
Carlton House, Commerce Way, Lancing, West Sussex
BN15 8TA
Tel: 0903 761100

George Solly Organisation Ltd.
111 Watlington Street,
Reading RE1 4RQ
Tel: 0734 566477

Suppliers of Essential Oils and Aromatherapy Products

House of Neroli at Oakelbrook Mill,
Newent, Glos. GL18 1HD
Tel: 0531 821875

J.M.R. Paramedical Products (Yorkshire),
17 Rossett Holt Close,
Harrogate, Yorkshire HG2 9AD
Tel: 0423 505707

Index

Abductor muscles 21
Accounting 196
Acne 81
Actinic ray 143
Adductor muscles 21
Adipose tissue 78
Adrenal gland 47, 72, 74, 75
  hormones of 74
Adrenalin 47, 74
Andrenocorticotropic hormone 72
Aerated bath 118
  treatment 119
Agote, Louis 38
Air 59–62
  exhalation of 62
  inspiration of 62
  intake of 61
Alopecia areata 82
Alveolar tissue 81
Alveoli 59, 61
Amino acids 57
Amp
  explanation of 129
Anaemia 36
  pernicious 36
  simple 36
Anatomy
  relationship with physiology 3
Anatomy and Physiology
  glossary of terminology 7, 91
  of the heart 3
  history 4–6
Anus 55
Appendicitis 58
Arachnoid 42
Arm
  bones of 12
  muscles of 20, 25
Arterial system 31, 32
Arteriosclerosis 38
Atherosclerosis 38
Atrium—right and left 30
Auditory nerve 80
Auditory ossicles 80
Autonomic neurological system 40, 46, 48
  parts of 46
Axon 40

Bell's palsy 49
Bile 57
Bladder 65, 66, 67, 68
Blood 33
  constituent parts 34
  from mother to unborn child 69

transfusions 38
types 34
Blue baby 38
Body massage 105–6
Bone articulations 8–11
  amphiarthroses 10
  ball and socket 10
  gliding joints 10
  hinge 10
  pivot 10
  synarthroses 10
Bones 8
  cavity within 84
  composition of 8
  distribution of 11
  fractures 15–16
  functions of 8
  hyoid bone 14
  joint articulations 8–11
  of the arm 12
  of the foot 13–14
  of the hand 13
  of the leg 13
  of the pelvis 13
  of the shoulder girdle 12
  of the skull 11–12
  of the spine 12
  of the thorax 12
  types of 8
Brain 42
  anatomy of 42, 46
Breasts 81
  hormonal activity 81
Bright, Dr. Richard 70
Bright's disease 69
Bronchial tubes 59
Bronchitis 63
Bronchioles 59, 61
Bursitis 11

Caecum 54
Calcium balance 74
Capsules of Bowman 67
Carbohydrates 57
Cardiac muscle 19
Cardiac oedema 89
Cortico-steroids 74
Cataract 82
Central neurological system 40
Cerebellum 42, 43
  function of 43
Cerebrum 42–43
  functions of 43
Cervicitis 69

Cervix 66
Choroid 78, 79
Chromosomes 85
Clinic premises 193–4
  fire extinguishers 194
  first aid provisions 194
  insurance 194
  licence 194
  planning consent 193
  temperature 194
  toilet facilities 194
Clitoris 66
Collagen 85, 89
Colon
  ascending 55
  descending 55
  sigmoid 55
  transverse 55
Combined treatments 109
Conjunctivitis 82
Connective tissue 86, 89
  adipose 86
  areolar 86
  bone 86
  cartilage 86
  fibrous 86
  muscular 87
  nervous 87
Convoluted tubules 67
Cornea 78, 79
Couches 198–201
Cramp 28
Cranial nerves 44–5
Cretinism 73, 75
Cupping 104–5
Cystitis 69

Deincrustation 139, 141
Dendrites 40
Dermis 77, 78
Diabetes mellitus 75
Diaphragm 59–61
Diathermic epilation 158–9
Digestive system 4, 51–8
  conditions and diseases of 58
  function of 51–52
Digestive tract 52
  movement of food 57
  organs of 52
Direct current equipment 132
  type and care of batteries 132
Disaccharides 57
Diseases
  of the skeleton 16–17
  of the muscular system 27–8
  of the vascular system 36, 38
DNA 85
Ductless glands 72
Duodenum 53, 56

Dura mater 42
Dwarfism 72

Ear 79–80
  glossary of terminology 84
  structures of 79
Ear drum 79, 80
Ectoderm 85
Eczema 82
Effleurage 100–1
Effluvation 156
Electrical energy 129–33
  measurements of 129
  medical currents 132–42
  principles of 129–30
  safety precautions 131–2
Electrical fuses 131
Electrical wiring 130
  colour coding 130
Electrology 158
Electro-magnetic spectrum 143–4
Endoblast 86
Endocrine glands 72
Endocrine system 4, 72–6
  terminology of 76
Enzymes 53
Epiblast 85
Epidermis 77, 78
Epiglottis 62
Epithelium 86
  simple 86
  stratified 86
Ergosterol 144
Erector pili muscles 78
Eustachian tube 80
Exercise 150–155
  benefits from 150
  mechanical equipment 154
  purpose of 150
  routine of 150
Exophthalmic goitre 74
Expenses 195
Extensor muscles 21
External ear 79, 80
  parts of 79
  purpose of 80
  secretions of 79
Eyes 78–79
  diseases and conditions of 82
  glossary of terminology 84
  structure of 78–79

Facial paralysis 49
Fallopian tubes 65
Faradic current 132, 133
  instrument types 134–6
  method of operation 136
  output required 133–4
  pad placement 133, 137–9

pad types 134
primary use for 133
summary of treatment 139
surge rate 136
treatment time 136–37
Fats 57
Fatty acids 57
Fibrositis 27
Finsen, Niels 144
Flexor muscles 21
Foam bath 118, 119
treatment 119
Food
body needs of 52
Foot
bones of 13–14
muscles of 26
Fractures
types of 15–16
Fulguration treatment 157–8
Fundus 66

Gall bladder 56
Galvanic current 132, 140
unit of measurement 140
Galvanic treatment 139–42
contra-indications to 142
deincrustation 141
iontophoretic 140–41
Gastric juice 53
Gene 85
Genito-urinary system 4, 65
conditions and diseases of 69–70
glossary of terminology 71
parts of 65
Gigantism 72
Glands of the body 72–5, 78
Glossary of terminology of the
accessory organs 84
anatomy and physiology 7
endocrine system 76
general medical 91–3
genito-urinary system 71
histology 90
muscular system 29
neurological system 49
respiratory system 64
skeletal system 18
vascular system 39
Glycerol 57
Goitre 75
Gonads 74
hormones of 75
of the female 75
of the male 75
Gonadotropic hormone 72
Gowns 204
Ground substance 85, 89
Gyrator massagers 107–9

precautions with 109

Hacking 102–3
Hand
bones of 13
muscles of 25
Head and neck
muscles of 22–3
Haemoglobin
carboxy- 33
oxy- 33
Haemophilia 37
Heart
anatomy 3, 30
cavities of 31
chambers of 30
circulatory systems of 31
effect of vasopressin 72
physiology 3, 30
Heartburn 58
Heat treatment
contra-indications to 113
equipment and methods 113–20
principal effect of 112–13
High frequency 156–8
treatment categories 156–7
Histology 85–91
glossary of terminology 90
History of anatomy and physiology 4–6
Hordeolum 82
Housemaid's knee 11
Hyoid bone 14
Hyperaemia 148
Hypophysis 72
Hypothalamus 46

Ileo-caecal valve 54
Ileum 53, 54
Infrared ray 143, 147–9
benefits from 147–9
contra-indications to 149
treatment 149
Insulin 56, 75
Insurance 194
premises and contents 194
professional public indemnity 194
third party indemnity 194
Interferential currents 159
Internal ear 80
parts of 80
purpose of 80
Intestine
large 52, 54
small 52, 53
Interstitial substance 85
Involuntary muscle 19
Iontophoresis 139
equipment for treatment 140
Iris 78–9

Islets of Langerhans   56, 75

Jaundice   58
Jejunum   53

Keloids   82
Kidneys   66–7
  effects of vasopressin   72
  principal parts   66
  results of kidney function   68
Kidney stones   69
Kneading   101–2
Koch, Robert   63

Lachrymal glands   79
Lactation   81
Lactiferous sinuses   81
Landsteiner, Karl   34, 35, 38
Large intestine   54–5
  parts of 54
  position of   55
Larynx   52
Leg
  bones of   13
  muscles of   25
Leucocytes   34
Leukaemia   37
Licence to practise   194
Light spectrum   143
Ling, Henreich   98
Liver   52, 56, 57
  cirrhosis of 58
  lobes of   56
Lower, Richard   38
Lumbago   27
Lungs   59, 62
  capacity of   62
  effect of vasopressin   72
Lymph   36–37
  effect of vacuum suction on   123
Lymphatic duct   36
Lymphatic system   36–7
  of the breasts   81
Lymph nodes   36, 37
  of the intestine   54
Lymphocytes   36

Macrocytes   37
Mammary areola   81
Mammary glands   81
  effect of oxytocin   72
Massage   97–11
  contra-indications to 109–10
  glossary of terminology   111
  history of   97–98
  mechanical   107–9
  Swedish   98–106
Mastoid antrum   80

Mechanical massage   107–9
  types of   107
Medullated nerve   41
Medulla oblongata   42, 43
  anatomy and physiology of   43
  function of   43
  relationship with spinal cord   44
Melanin   144
Membranes   89
Meninges   42
Menstrual cycle   65, 68–9
Mesoblast   85
Mesoderm   85
Metabolic hormones   72
Microwave   159
Middle ear   80
  purpose of   80
Mitosis   85, 89
Monosaccharides   57
Mucous bursae   11
Mucous membrane   89
Muscle
  diseases of 27–8
  energy utilisation   20
  excretion of waste products   20–1
  fuel supply   20
  groups of   21
  points of attachment to bone   19–20
  reaction to temperature   26
  types of   19, 20
Muscles
  of the arms   20, 21, 25
  of the back   24
  of the body   22–3
  of the head and neck   22–3
  of the legs   25–7
  of the stomach   53
  of the trunk   24–25
Muscular system   4, 19
  glossary of terminology   29
Myeline   40

Nail   78
Nasal pharynx
  relationship to middle ear   80
Nephrites   70
Nerve cell   40
  composite parts   40
Nerves
  cranial   44
  mixed   44
  motor or efferent   44
  sensory or afferent   44, 78
  spinal   45
Nerve stimulus   20
Neuralgia   49
Neurological system   4, 40–50
  glossary of terminology   50
  diseases of   49

divisions of   40
  parts of   44
Neuron   40
  composite parts   40
  within brain   42
Newton, Isaac 143
Nose   59
  relationship with lachrymal glands   79
Nucleotides   85

Oedema   89
  help in reduction   123–4
Oesophagus   52, 53
  lining   53
Oestrogen   65, 75
Oils for massage, choice of 106–7
Oil massage   106
Optic nerve endings   79
  receptor   79
  sensory   79
Ovaries   65, 72, 75
Ovum   65
  expelling of   69
Oxytocin hormone   72

Pancreas   52, 56, 72, 75
Papillae
  filliform   52
  fungiform   52
  vallate   52
Paraffin wax   117
Parasympathetic nerve system   46
  effects of   46
  parts of   46
Parathormone   74
Parathyroid glands   72, 74
Parietal layer   62
Parkinson's disease   49
Patient assessment   189–92
  general observation   189
  of weight   190
Patient's record card   189
Patient support   206–8
Pelvic bones   8
Pelvis
  bones of   13
Penis   66
Pepsin   53
Peptones   57
Percussor massagers   107
Peripheral nerves   44
  types of   44
Peristalsis   57
Pétrissage   101, 103
Peyer's patches   54
Phagocytes   34
Pharynx   53
  openings into   53
Phosphorus balance   74

Physiology
  relationship with anatomy   3
Pia mater   42
Pituitary gland   46, 72
  hormones of   72
Placenta   69
Planning consent   193
Plasma   34
Platelets   34
Pleura   62
Pleural cavity   62
Pleurisy   63
Pneumoconiosis   63
Poliomyelitis   28
Polypeptides   57
Polysaccharides   57
Pons varoli   46
Professional ethics   205–6
Professionalism   205
Progesterone   65, 75
Pronator muscles   21
Prostate gland   68
Proteins   57
Psoriasis   82
Ptyalin   52
Pulmonary circulation   31
Pulmonary system   61
Pulmonary tuberculosis   63
Pupil   79
  method of controlling light   79
Pyloric valve
  function of   57
Pyrosis   58

Radiant heat   143, 147
Radiant heat bath   120
  expense of running   130
Rectum   55
Reflex action   48–9
Registration of business name   193
Rennin   53
Reproductive cycle   69
Respiratory passages   61
  upper   60
Respiratory system   4, 59
  conditions and diseases of   63
  glossary of terminology   64
  parts of   59
Respiratory tract
  lower   59
  upper   59
Retina   79
Rib cage   8
Ringworm—of the scalp   83
Roman baths   112, 113
Rotator muscles   21
Rugae
  of the stomach   53

Salivary glands   52
 secretions of   52
 types of   52
Saturation high frequency treatment   157
Sauna bath   112, 115–17
 expense of running   129–30
 treatment   116–17
Scales   201–2
Sclera   78, 79
Sciatica 49
Scrotum   66
Sclerosis   28
Sebaceous glands   78
Semen   68, 69
Sensory nerve endings   78
Septum   30
Serous membrane   89
Sex glands   74
Sex organs
 effect of thymus gland   74
Sinusoidal current   132
Skeletal system   4, 8–17
 diseases of   16–17
 glossary of terminology   18
Skin   77–8
 diseases and conditions of 81, 82, 83
 functions of   77
 glossary of terminology   84
 relationship with excretory system   69
 structure of   77, 78
Skull   8, 10, 11
 bones of   11
Slimming
 effect of vacuum sunction   123
 record cards   189
Stye   82
Somatotropic hormone   72
Spark treatment   156–7
Spermatozoon   69, 85
Sphincter muscles   21
Spinal column   8
 bones of   12
 curvature of   14–15
Spinal cord   44
 anatomy and physiology of   44
 position of   45
Spinal curvature
 causes of   14
 types of   14–15
Spinal nerves   45
Starches   57
Steam bath   112, 113–14
 expense of running   129–30
 treatment   113–14
Sterilisers   203
Stomach   52, 57
 coverings of   53
 curvature of   53
 muscles of   53

 parts of   53
Succus entericus   54
Sudoriferous glands   78
Sun-ray   143, 144
Supinator muscle   21
Supra-renal gland   74
Sweat glands   78
 apocrine   78
 eccrine   78
Swedish massage   98–106
 exercise for efficient hand movement   105
 movements   100–5
Sympathetic nerve system   46
 effects of   46
 parts of   46
Sympatheticotonic type person
 reasons for   48
Synovial fluid   11
Synovial membrane   89
Synovitis   11
System circulation   31
Systems of the body   3–4
 lymphatic   36
 neurological   40
 vascular   30

Talc massage—*see Swedish massage*
Tapotement   101
Tax relief   193
Tear glands   79
Teeth   52
 types of   52
Tesla, Nicolai   156
Testes   65, 66, 72, 75
Testosterone   75
Tetany   74
Thermal baths   112
Thoracic duct   35, 57
Thorax
 bones of   12
 position of lungs within   60
Thymus gland   72, 75
Thyroid gland   72–4
 effect on activity   73, 75
 secretions from   73
Thyrotropic hormone   72
Thyroxine   72
Tineacapitas   83
Tongue   52
 papillae of 52
Torticollis   27
Towels   204
Toxins, elimination of   112
Trachea   61, 73
Treatment oils   125
Treatment trolleys   201
Trio-iodothyronine   73
 effects of over secretion   74
 effects of under secretion   73

Trunk
  muscles of   24–25
Turkish baths   113–14
Tympanic membrane   79, 80
Tympanum   80

Ultrasound   175–85
  effects of   176–7
  measurement of   180–81
  method of treatment   178–80
Ultraviolet ray   143–7
  contra-indications to   147
  cosmetic radiation range   144
  equipment   144
  factors relating to exposure times   146
  germicidal radiation range   144
  in diagnosis   144
  method of treatment   145–6
  protection for eyes   146
  unit of measurement   143
Umbilical cord   69
Uniform   205
Ureter   65, 67–8
Urethra   65
Urinary bladder   65
Urine   67–8
  amount produced   67
  composition of   68
  retention   68
Uterus   65
  effect of oxytocin   72
  relationship in reproductive cycle   69

Vacuum suction treatment   121–8
  conditions benefiting from   124, 128
  contra-indications of   124

effect of   123–4
  equipment   121–3
  history of   121
  measurement of vacuum   122, 125–7
  method of treatment   125
  selection of cup size   125–8
Vagina   66
Vagotonic type person
  reasons for   48
Valvulae conniventes   54
Varicose veins   37
  benefit from vacuum massage   125
  causes of   37
Vascular system   4, 30, 33
  conditions, deficiencies and diseases of   36
  glossary of terminology   39
Vasopressin hormone   72
Venous system   31
Ventricles—right and left   30
Vermiform appendix   54
Verruca   83
Villi   54
Visceral layer   62
Vitamin D   144
volt, explanation of   129
Voluntary muscle   19
Vulva   66

Warts   83
Watt, explanation of   129
Wax baths   117–18
  treatment   117–18
Weight assessment   166–7
Weiner, A.S.   35
Wry neck   27